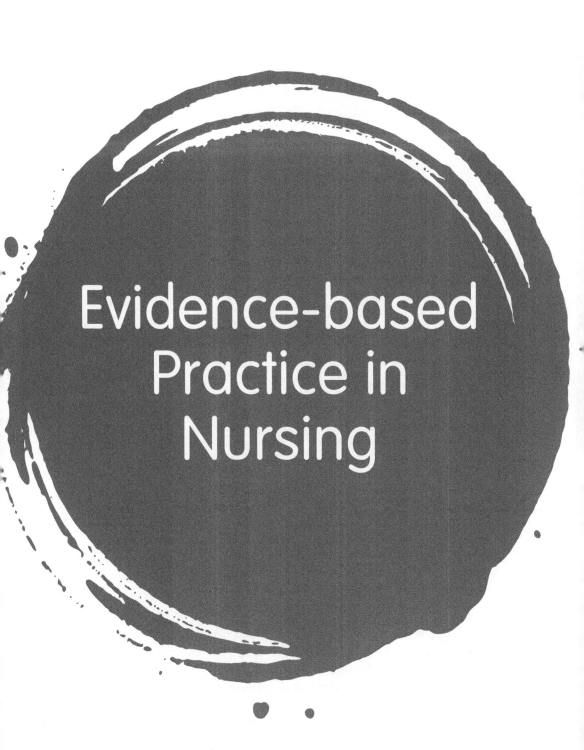

Evidence-based Practice in Nursing

Sara Miller McCune founded SAGE Publishing in 1965 to support the dissemination of usable knowledge and educate a global community. SAGE publishes more than 1000 journals and over 800 new books each year, spanning a wide range of subject areas. Our growing selection of library products includes archives, data, case studies and video. SAGE remains majority owned by our founder and after her lifetime will become owned by a charitable trust that secures the company's continued independence.

Los Angeles | London | New Delhi | Singapore | Washington DC | Melbourne

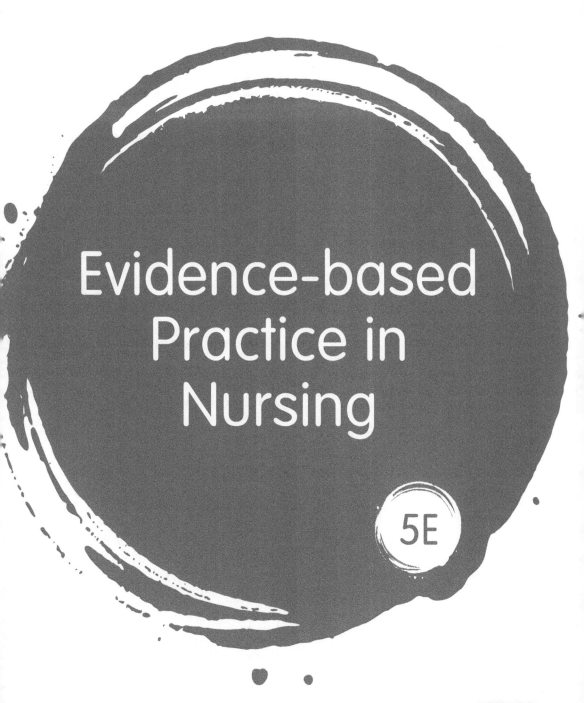

Evidence-based Practice in Nursing

5E

Peter Ellis

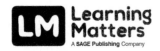

Learning Matters
A SAGE Publishing Company
1 Oliver's Yard
55 City Road
London EC1Y 1SP

SAGE Publications Inc.
2455 Teller Road
Thousand Oaks, California 91320

SAGE Publications India Pvt Ltd
B 1/I 1 Mohan Cooperative Industrial Area
Mathura Road
New Delhi 110 044

SAGE Publications Asia-Pacific Pte Ltd
3 Church Street
#10-04 Samsung Hub
Singapore 049483

Editor: Laura Walmsley
Development editor: Richenda Milton-Daws
Senior project editor: Chris Marke
Marketing manager: Ruslana Khatagova
Cover design: Sheila Tong
Typeset by: C&M Digitals (P) Ltd, Chennai, India
Printed in the UK

Library of Congress Control Number: 2022940645

British Library Cataloguing in Publication Data

A catalogue record for this book is available from
the British Library

ISBN 978-1-5297-7971-4
ISBN 978-1-5297-7970-7 (pbk)

At SAGE we take sustainability seriously. Most of our products are printed in the UK using responsibly sourced
papers and boards. When we print overseas we ensure sustainable papers are used as measured by the PREPS
grading system. We undertake an annual audit to monitor our sustainability.

Contents

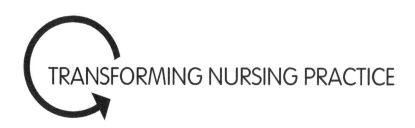

TRANSFORMING NURSING PRACTICE

Transforming Nursing Practice is a series tailor made for pre-registration students nurses. Each book in the series is:

 Affordable

 Mapped to the NMC Standards of proficiency for registered nurses

 Full of active learning features

 Focused on applying theory to practice

Each book addresses a core topic and they have been carefully developed to be simple to use, quick to read and written in clear language.

An invaluable series of books that explicitly relates to the NMC standards. Each book covers a different topic that students need to explore in order to develop into a qualified nurse... I would recommend this series to all Pre-Registered nursing students whatever their field or year of study.

LINDA ROBSON,
Senior Lecturer at Edge Hill University

Many titles in the series are on our recommended reading list and for good reason - the content is up to date and easy to read. These are the books that actually get used beyond training and into your nursing career.

EMMA LYDON,
Adult Student Nursing

ABOUT THE SERIES EDITORS

DR MOOI STANDING is an Independent Nursing Consultant (UK and International) and is responsible for the core knowledge, adult nursing and personal and professional learning skills titles. She is an experienced NMC Quality Assurance Reviewer of educational programmes and a Professional Regulator Panellist on the NMC Practice Committee. Mooi is also Board member of Special Olympics Malaysia, enabling people with intellectual disabilities to participate in sports and athletics nationally and internationally.

DR SANDRA WALKER is a Clinical Academic in Mental Health working between Southern Health Trust and the University of Southampton and responsible for the mental health nursing titles. She is a Qualified Mental Health Nurse with a wide range of clinical experience spanning more than 25 years.

BESTSELLING TEXTBOOKS

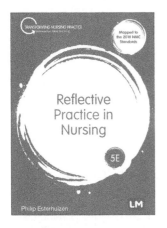

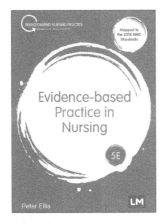

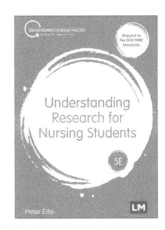

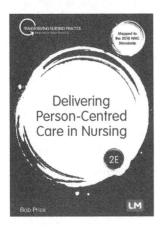

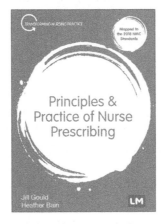

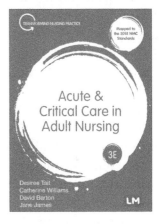

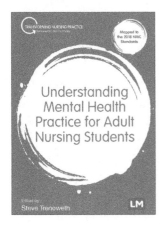

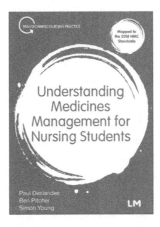

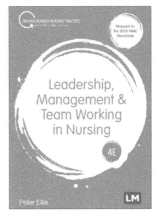

You can find a full list of textbooks in the *Transforming Nursing Practice* series at
https://uk.sagepub.com/TNP-series

Foreword

The Transforming Nursing Practice series includes several titles that focus on personal and professional learning skills needed by nurses in order to deliver safe and effective care. *Evidence-based Practice in Nursing* is a key text in this respect. The reader is encouraged to develop specific personal qualities ('dispositions of the evidence-based nurse'), including being a questioning, critical and creative thinker, reflective and reflexive, morally active, self-aware and considerate of others. The book argues that cultivating these important qualities goes hand in hand with the development and application of professional knowledge and skills in evidence-based nursing. The reader is shown how different types of evidence (research, practical knowledge/experience, health policy, patient preferences, ethical or legal issues and interprofessional feedback) can be identified, evaluated and applied to inform and enhance the quality of nursing care. This is reinforced in each chapter with reference to the relevant NMC standards of proficiency for registered nurses. The book's relevance to the practicalities of delivering high-quality, patient-centred care is highlighted in many interesting and varied case studies. They are invaluable in enabling nursing students to apply evidence-based practice within adult and children's learning disabilities and mental health fields of nursing. Readers' understanding of evidence-based practice in nursing is continually tested by a range of challenging learning activities. After reading this book, nursing students, registered nurses and others will have a very good grasp of the complex nature of evidence-based practice, and how they can incorporate these principles and processes to enhance the care that they give to patients.

In the fifth edition of this very popular book, the authors have incorporated changes that take account of new developments, reviewer comments and readers' feedback. These include: a) updating and adding new references, further reading and informative websites to encourage readers to consider the evidence behind the material presented in each chapter; b) refining frameworks and guidance in writing research critiques; c) incorporating research studies linking evidence-based practice to the Coronavirus pandemic; and d) presenting additional learning activities to help readers develop critical thinking skills and apply them to their evidence-based practice. Hence, in updating the book, the authors mirror how evidence-based practice is constantly evolving in response to new research findings, health policy and feedback from service users. This reinforces the need for lifelong learning and professional development, continually refreshing the knowledge and skills described to deliver high-quality, evidence-based nursing practice. The book is therefore an excellent resource both for nursing students in preparing for registration, and for registered nurses when critically reflecting on their clinical practice for the purposes of NMC revalidation.

Dr Mooi Standing

Series Editor

About the authors

Peter Ellis is an independent nursing and health and social care writer and consultant, and CEO of Intelligent Care Software. Peter was most recently a Registered Manager and Nursing Director in the Hospice and social care settings. Prior to this, he was a senior lecturer and programme director at Canterbury Christ Church University where he taught understanding research, among other topics, to undergraduate and postgraduate nursing students. Peter is also an Honorary Senior Research Fellow of Canterbury Christ Church University and has a special interest, including ongoing research, in palliative and end-of-life care.

Contributors

Dr Mooi Standing is an Independent Nursing Consultant (UK and International) and is responsible for the core knowledge, adult nursing and personal and professional learning skills titles. She is an experienced NMC Quality Assurance Reviewer of educational programmes and a Professional Regulator Panellist on the NMC Practice Committee. Mooi is also a Board member of Special Olympics Malaysia, enabling people with intellectual disabilities to participate in sports and athletics nationally and internationally.

Dr Caroline Thomas is a Senior Lecturer in Education and a researcher in the School of Education at Canterbury Christ Church University. She is also a Nursing and Midwifery Council Quality Assurance Reviewer for midwifery and nursing practice.

Acknowledgements

For ERE and HJE using evidence and understanding in their work to make the world a better place.

Introduction

One of the enduring tensions of nursing is the theory–practice gap. Some nurses regard this as an inevitable consequence of degree-level nursing in the UK where academics are seen as being far removed from the realities of practice, while some academics regard this as being a result of practising nurses' hesitance to engage in degree-level education.

Whatever the reality of the theory–practice gap, the conscientious adoption of a coherent framework for the progression of practice through engagement with personal development and new sources of information, while maintaining a view on the realities of clinical nursing, might well help solve this dilemma for practising professionals.

In this book, we take the view that the purpose of academic nursing is to support the enhancement of practice. To achieve this, it is necessary for academic nursing to take account of the nature and realities of clinical practice. To this end, we present a view of evidence-based practice that is both grounded in academic nursing (information, knowledge, evidence) and practical nursing (experience, reflection, reflexivity and patient preference). What seems clear to us in presenting this argument is that nursing is a practical undertaking, and we cannot and should not engage in the creation of evidence that does not support this.

The subsequent sections will enable you to gain an overview of the messages contained within the book and how these might fit together to inform your development as an action-oriented evidence-driven nurse.

Chapter 1: What is evidence-based nursing? This introductory chapter sets the scene for the rest of the book and demonstrates how the various strands of evidence may be drawn together to create an inclusive picture of evidence-based nursing practice. It also examines some of the dispositions and characteristics that it might be necessary for a nurse to adopt in order to become truly evidence-based.

Chapter 2: Sources of knowledge for evidence-based care. Access to information is easier now than it has ever been. The internet provides nurses with access to sources of information that are both immediate and accessible. Newspapers, television, journals and other media carry stories about issues that affect not only health, but the ways in which healthcare is delivered. The novice nurse may be tempted to use these sources of information in an unquestioning way, readily accepting what they say as being applicable to nursing practice. The more experienced nurse or student may feel that other sources of information are more appropriate – for instance, nursing journals and professional internet-based nursing resources.

While more faith can be placed in professional sources of information, we argue in this book that there remains a need to show some caution in the sourcing and interpretation of sources of knowledge, and that even the best sources of information for practice require that the evidence-based nurse applies some criteria to judge the truth and usefulness of the information these sources contain.

Chapter 3: Critiquing research: general points. Any book about evidence-based practice (EBP) cannot ignore the contribution of research to the nursing evidence base. Unlike many other books about EBP, this book regards research as being of only equal importance as other sources of knowledge. Chapter 3 will explore methods for critiquing the elements of research that appear in all research papers.

Chapter 4: Critiquing research: approach-specific elements. This is a continuation of Chapter 3 and seeks to expand upon the critiquing of research that is undertaken in either the qualitative or quantitative paradigm. The Appendix to this book, which is a critiquing framework, should be read alongside Chapters 3 and 4, as together they are intended to provide guidance of the critiquing of research for either academic purposes or to inform practice.

Chapter 5: Making sense of subjective experience. A fundamental aspect of being able to draw on many sources of information at once and to make sense of what one is hearing and seeing is having the ability to be both reflective and reflexive. Rather than explain how these strategies are practised (which is explored in the book *Reflective Practice in Nursing* in this series), Chapter 5 examines how they can contribute to our understanding of sources of evidence other than research – namely, subjective knowledge.

Chapter 6: Working with others to achieve evidence-based care. Here, we explore collaborative working as a strategy for improving our evidence base for practice. The chapter explores how we as nurses can use others to develop ourselves and our understanding of care delivery. Working with others means working with different health and social care professionals (which is explored in the book *Nursing and Collaborative Practice*, also in this series) and, most importantly, patients themselves. Evidence-based practice requires nurses to be aware of, respond to and engage with the input of all individuals involved with an episode of care.

Chapter 7: Clinical decision-making in evidence-based nursing. This chapter considers how the nurse might draw together various sources of evidence, reconcile the various influences on practice and apply the skills identified in earlier chapters in order to make worthwhile clinical decisions with individual patients. It challenges the reader to think about the ethical context of their decisions and how these affect individual patients. It also draws together the threads of the arguments presented in the other chapters, and creates a practical guide to evaluate clinical decision-making. (The issues identified in this chapter are explored in more depth in *Clinical Judgement and Decision-Making in Nursing*, also in this series.)

Chapter 8: Using evidence in the workplace. Here we explore some mechanisms by which evidence may be translated into meaningful practice. This chapter examines the social, practical and human barriers to the use of evidence in practice. It examines barriers to change and how change management strategies might be used to overcome these. It concentrates on personal and team strategies to support the adoption of evidence and what benefits might accrue from these.

Requirements from the NMC Standards

Evidence-based nursing requires the nurse to have knowledge and skills, which are outlined in detail in the document *Future Nurse: Standards of Proficiency for Registered Nurses* (NMC, 2018a). These Standards are used by educational institutions when planning professional courses. They are grouped into seven 'Platforms', as shown in the box below.

NMC Future Nurse: Standards of Proficiency for Registered Nurses

- **Platform 1: Being an accountable professional**

Registered nurses act in the best interests of people, putting them first and providing nursing care that is person-centred, safe and compassionate. They act professionally at all times and use their knowledge and experience to make evidence-based decisions about care. They communicate care effectively, are role models for others, and are accountable for their actions. Registered nurses continually reflect on their practice and keep abreast of new and emerging developments in nursing, health and care.

- **Platform 2: Promoting health and preventing ill health**

Registered nurses play a key role in improving and maintaining the mental, physical and behavioural health and well-being of people, families, communities and populations. They support and enable people at all stages of life and in all care settings to make informed choices about how to manage health challenges in order to maximise their quality of life and improve health outcomes. They are actively involved in the prevention of and protection against disease and ill health, and engage in public health, community development and global health agendas, and in the reduction of health inequalities.

- **Platform 3: Assessing needs and planning care**

Registered nurses prioritise the needs of people when assessing and reviewing their mental, physical, cognitive, behavioural, social and spiritual needs. They use information obtained

(Continued)

during assessments to identify the priorities and requirements for person-centred and evidence-based nursing interventions and support. They work in partnership with people to develop person-centred care plans that take into account their circumstances, characteristics and preferences.

- **Platform 4: Providing and evaluating care**

Registered nurses take the lead in providing evidence-based, compassionate and safe nursing interventions. They ensure that the care they provide and delegate is person-centred and of a consistently high standard. They support people of all ages in a range of care settings. They work in partnership with people, families and carers to evaluate whether care is effective and the goals of care have been met in line with their wishes, preferences and desired outcomes.

- **Platform 5: Leading and managing nursing care and working in teams**

Registered nurses provide leadership by acting as a role model for best practice in the delivery of nursing care. They are responsible for managing nursing care and are accountable for the appropriate delegation and supervision of care provided by others in the team, including lay carers. They play an active and equal role in the interdisciplinary team, collaborating and communicating effectively with a range of colleagues.

- **Platform 6: Improving safety and quality of care**

Registered nurses make a key contribution to the continuous monitoring and quality improvement of care and treatment in order to enhance health outcome and people's experience of nursing and related care. They assess risks to safety or experience and take appropriate action to manage those, putting the best interests, needs and preferences of people first.

- **Platform 7: Coordinating care**

Registered nurses play a leadership role in coordinating and managing the complex nursing and integrated care needs of people at any stage of their lives, across a range of organisations and settings. They contribute to processes of organisational change through an awareness of local and national policies.

This book draws from these Standards and presents the relevant ones at the beginning of each chapter.

Learning features

Learning from reading text is not always easy. Therefore, to provide variety and to assist with the development of independent learning skills and the application of theory to practice, this book contains activities, example stories, scenarios (some with questions), case studies, concept summaries, further reading and useful websites to enable you to participate in your own learning. You will need to develop your own study skills and 'learn how to learn' to get the best from the material. The book cannot provide all the answers, but instead provides a framework for your learning.

The activities in the book will help you in particular to make sense of, and learn about, the material being presented. Some activities ask you to reflect on aspects of practice, or your experience of it, or the people or situations you encounter. *Reflection* is an essential skill in nursing, and it helps you to understand the world around you and often to identify how things might be improved. Other activities will help you develop key graduate skills, such as your ability to *think critically* about a topic in order to challenge received wisdom, or your ability to *research a topic and find appropriate information and evidence*, and to be able to *make decisions* using that evidence in situations that are often difficult and time-pressured. Communication and working as part of a team are core to all nursing practice, and some activities will ask you to think about your *communication skills* to help develop these.

All the activities require you to take a break from reading the text, think through the issues presented and carry out some independent study, possibly using the internet. Where appropriate, there are sample answers presented at the end of each chapter, and these will help you to understand more fully your own reflections and independent study. You will gain most from the activities if you try to complete them yourself before reading the suggested answers. Remember, academic study will always require independent work; attending lectures will never be enough to be successful on your programme, and these activities will help to deepen your knowledge and understanding of the issues under scrutiny and give you practice at working on your own.

You might want to think about completing these activities as part of your personal development plan (PDP) or portfolio. After completing the activity, write it up in your PDP or portfolio in a section devoted to that particular skill, then look back over time to see how far you have developed. You can also do more of the activities for a key skill in which you have identified a weakness, and this will help build your skill and confidence in this area.

There is a Glossary of terms at the end of the book that provides an interpretation of some of the terminology in the context of the subject of the book. Glossary terms are in **bold** the first time they appear.

All chapters have further reading and useful websites listed at the end, with notes to show you why we think they will be helpful to you. The websites will also help you to remain up to date with developments in this aspect of practice as awareness of key issues grows and policies develop.

We hope that you find this book helpful in developing your professional practice, and that it challenges you to ensure you provide care and support that reduces the risk of vulnerability and promotes dignity, respect and a positive quality of life.

Chapter 1 · What is evidence-based nursing?

Peter Ellis

NMC Future Nurse: Standards of Proficiency for Registered Nurses

This chapter will address the following platforms and proficiencies:

Platform 1: Being an accountable professional

At the point of registration, the registered nurse will be able to:

1.8 demonstrate the knowledge, skills and ability to think critically when applying evidence and drawing on experience to make evidence informed decisions in all situations.

1.9 understand the need to base all decisions regarding care and interventions on people's needs and preferences, recognising and addressing any personal and external factors that may unduly influence their decisions.

Platform 3: Assessing needs and planning care

At the point of registration, the registered nurse will be able to:

3.4 understand and apply a person-centred approach to nursing care, demonstrating shared assessment, planning, decision making and goal setting when working with people, their families, communities and populations of all ages.

3.5 demonstrate the ability to accurately process all information gathered during the assessment process to identify needs for individualised nursing care and develop person-centred evidence-based plans for nursing interventions with agreed goals.

Chapter aims

....

After reading this chapter, you will be able to:

* understand what evidence for nursing practice is;
* identify the key components of evidence;
* understand why evidence for practice is important;
* start to develop an understanding of critical practice.

Introduction

Nurses work in ever-changing environments of care. Changes in national and local policy and guidelines, improvements in technology and pharmaceuticals, the changing demography of the world and developments in society all impact on the ways in which we deliver care. Not only do we face the challenge of a constantly evolving workplace, but as a student nurse you have to try to make sense of what you learn in the classroom and how this relates to the realities of what you experience in the workplace. As a staff nurse, the pressures increase somewhat as you continue to work in the ever-changing environment, one that requires you to evolve and develop with it in order to deliver high-quality care, for which you are now professionally accountable and where you must act as a practice supervisor and role model to nursing students.

The pressures of care delivery can lead to an overwhelming feeling of helplessness. Perhaps you feel that you might not know all you think you should know before you go on to the wards, or that what you have learnt might well be out of date soon. Being prepared for life as a nurse requires you to embrace the many opportunities for lifelong learning so you can develop skills in identifying and evaluating information (evidence) that will stand you in good stead throughout your nursing career.

This chapter sets the scene for the rest of the book by describing an attitude and approach to learning and development that will help support you, as a student or trained nurse, in making sense of where you work and what you do in practice. It aims to stimulate you to think about how and why you practise in the way you do and how you can make sense of the various influences on your practice.

If you think that evidence-based practice is all about the application of research, this chapter will challenge you to reconsider. In this book, we take the view that research is only one of the sources of knowledge and understanding that inform the evidence on which to base practice, and that it is the role of the nurse to understand, and apply, at least some of these sources.

We argue that, in order to truly act in an evidential way in practice, the nurse needs to knit together many sources of evidence. The position we take is that sources of knowledge may stand alone as evidence, or may serve to validate or refute other sources of evidence. For example, a randomised controlled trial may demonstrate the worth of a 'keep fit' intervention for weight loss, and this evidence may be validated by a qualitative enquiry that shows that the people involved enjoy the keep fit and want to do it – hence they do it and so lose weight. Conversely, they may not enjoy the process and therefore the intervention will ultimately fail even though, if they were to engage with the keep fit, they would lose weight.

In this book, we demonstrate that all the different sources of information and influences on the way in which nursing is practised are potentially of equal importance at one time or another. We further show that to nurse effectively in the twenty-first century, and beyond, requires you to be able to identify and use all forms of information in order to turn them into evidence that can inform practice. One of the big messages of this book is that information and knowledge are there to inform practice as part of a broader understanding of practice situations and the influences on what we as professionals and our patients believe and how we act.

In order to achieve this, this chapter explores some of the influences that have shaped nursing practice. It describes and examines the rise of evidence-based practice and develops a big-picture view of how you can prepare yourself for the challenges of modern nursing practice. Rising to this challenge requires you to adopt a constantly questioning approach to your practice that is both beneficial to your learning and working life, and, ultimately and importantly, to your patients – that is, to be a truly evidential practitioner you need to adopt a questioning and reflective attitude to your work.

Activity 1.1   Reflection

Try to remember what made you want to become a nurse in the first place. Stop and think about what you thought would inform and guide what you would do in your everyday practice as a nurse before you became a nursing student. Talk to others on your programme about what they felt or thought about this.

As this activity is based on your own observation, there is no outline answer at the end of the chapter.

The likely feeling you will have about Activity 1.1 is that your practice would be guided by the people who teach you and those who work with you in practice. Of course, this is widely the case, but there are a few issues with the apprenticeship model of nurse education in which matron or sister always knew best in that it can, unquestioned, propagate outdated or even poor practice. Sometimes teachers and mentors do not know the answers to questions, and even if they do, learning to be dependent on others for information and understanding is not the best way to prepare for life as an autonomous and evidence-based nurse. So, clearly developing a sense of the need for evidence to guide your own practice and the ability to identify and apply it early on in your career is no bad thing. What this means for nursing education is that it aims to teach you as much about how to think as it does about how to nurse. This is because nurses who are able to think, reflect and understand things for themselves are better equipped not only for the immediate challenges of practice, but also for the challenges and changes that are an inevitable part of future practice.

Why evidence-based nursing is important

There is an increasing culture of scrutiny of the work of health and social care professionals which has come about, at least in part, in response to various scandals (see the **case studies** below). Such public scandals have contributed to a climate of care in which nurses are increasingly required to be able to justify the decisions they make with and for patients. No longer is it good enough for nurses to claim they know what is best for their patients just because they are nurses. The rise in patient power and the governmental agenda of service user consultation and involvement – Department of Health (DH), 1989, 1991, 2001, 2012a; Medicines and Healthcare Products Regulatory Agency (MHRA), 2021; National Institute for Health and Care Excellence (NICE), 2011, 2013, 2022 – have created a climate of care in which nurses have to be able to justify not only what they do, but also how and why they are doing it.

Case studies: Scandals involving UK healthcare

On 25 February 2000, Victoria Climbié died after years of neglect and abuse from her aunt and aunt's boyfriend. In his report of the inquiry into the death of Victoria, Lord Laming (2003) states: *I found it hard to understand why established good medical practice, that would have undoubtedly helped clarify the complexities in Victoria's case, was not followed.*

In January 2001, the Redfern Report criticised the actions of a pathologist at the children's hospital, Alder Hey, for removing and retaining human organs and tissue samples without consent. The public outcry that followed led the UK government to publish new guidelines outlining the law on the handling of human body parts (**www.rlcinquiry.org.uk**).

On 15 April 2009, Margaret Haywood was struck off the Nursing and Midwifery Council's register for secretly filming the alleged neglect of elderly patients at the Royal Sussex Hospital. The public response to the programme had been one of outrage.

In 2013, the Francis Report into the failings at Mid Staffordshire NHS Foundation Trust made some important observations about the failure of care within the Trust.

The negative aspects of culture in the system were identified as including:

- *a lack of openness to criticism*
- *a lack of consideration for patients*
- *defensiveness*
- *looking inwards not outwards*
- *secrecy*
- *misplaced assumptions about the judgements and actions of others*
- *an acceptance of poor standards*
- *a failure to put the patient first in everything that is done.*

This report became one of the key drivers for change in care provision in the UK.

Orchid View in West Sussex was the scene of 19 unexplained deaths among its elderly residents. The chairman of the review into the failings at the care home, Nick Georgiou (West Sussex Adults Safeguarding Board, 2014), wrote: *What happened at Orchid View was more an avoidance of positive action to rectify problems, and a series of ineffectual action plans that were not acted on.*

Nursing takes place very much in the public eye, and when nurses and other health and social care professionals make mistakes, they come in for severe criticism. There is also a feeling in society at large that all care professionals should know what they are doing, why they are doing it and should do it well.

Such expectations are daunting but entirely understandable; most nurses aspire to live up to them. Clearly, knowledge of what evidence-based practice is will not be sufficient for you to meet these expectations; however, knowledge of how you might go about identifying evidence to inform practice and how you might subsequently assimilate this evidence into your practice will be. In short, evidence-based nursing practice is not an academic exercise; it is a means of knitting together knowledge from a number of different sources in a way that has the potential to impact positively on what we do as nurses: care.

Activity 1.2   Reflection

Think about a time when you, or a family member, were a patient. How well do you feel you were kept informed about the care you received and why it was being delivered in the way it was? Ask a more experienced colleague what it was like to be a nurse in the past and how the evidence-based care agenda has changed the way in which care is delivered. Do they think it is a good thing or a bad thing? Why?

An outline of what you might find is given at the end of the chapter.

Knowing what you are doing and why informs part of an important element of modern nursing and healthcare practice called **clinical governance**. Clinical governance is a system whereby what healthcare professionals do in practice is subjected to scrutiny to ensure that it is worthwhile, the correct policies and guidelines are in place, an audit of practice is happening and money is being spent wisely. NICE creates guidelines for how National Health Service (NHS) money is used. It uses evidence from many sources to inform the guidance produced, which is widely regarded as setting the standards for UK practice.

Activity 1.3   Evidence-based practice and research

Have a look at some NICE guidelines on a disease or other illness you know something about. Pay particular attention to what evidence informed the decision-making and who was involved in drawing up the guidance. Consider how you might gather the information you might need to answer the same question and whether you consider the approach taken by NICE to be comprehensive and reasonable.

The website address for NICE is given at the end of the chapter in the useful websites section.

As this activity is based on your own observation, there is no outline answer at the end of the chapter.

Not only is the requirement to evidence what we do as nurses a result of political and social pressure, but there are good moral reasons as to why nurses need to show that what they are doing is in the best interests of their patients. Accountability is a central tenet of the Nursing and Midwifery Council's *Code* (2018b), which states that nurses must:

Always practise in line with the best available evidence . . . To achieve this, you must:

6.1 make sure that any information or advice given is evidence-based, including information relating to using any healthcare products or services

6.2 maintain the knowledge and skills you need for safe and effective practice.

Beauchamp and Childress (2013) argue that ethical practice in healthcare requires that the providers of care, including nurses and student nurses, are mindful of what they term the four principles of healthcare ethics. These are:

- beneficence (doing good);
- non-maleficence (avoiding unnecessary harm);
- autonomy (respecting freedom of action);
- justice (fairness).

There are, of course, a number of other ethical approaches that might inform how we act as nurses, but the message from Beauchamp and Childress (2013) has clear connections as to why evidence is important in nursing. If we are to do good for our patients and avoid doing them harm, as well as supporting them to make choices about their care and then provide care in a consistent (fair) way, then we need to provide care which is based on evidence and not speculation, or the 'sister knows best' model discussed earlier.

The other main school of ethical thought, although there are many others (see *Understanding Ethics for Nursing Students*, also in this series), which might inform practice is that of consequentialism (doing things that have the best outcomes); the nurse might select a course of action with his or her patient that is perceived to have the highest probability of achieving the desired outcome of care.

In the UK, we are used to the idea that healthcare is provided 'free at the point of use'; indeed, this is one of the founding principles of the National Health Service, and one of the things that makes it such a special institution in which people hold great pride. However, 'free at the point of use' is not the same as 'free'. The money that funds the activity of the NHS comes directly out of the public purse; it is money that is raised through taxation and National Insurance contributions and, as such, it is money that needs to be spent wisely. There are many pressures on how NHS money is used, and to spend money on futile practices means there is less money available elsewhere in the system. The use of evidence in practice is therefore essential in order to help make the money available go as far as it can reasonably be expected to. The idea of getting good value for money links strongly to the principles of ethics and governance discussed above.

Some of the reasons why adopting an evidential approach to nursing is important are:

- accountability to our professional body;
- it improves the likelihood of good quality outcomes of care;
- professionalism of nursing;
- governance;
- it shows good use of resources;
- moral and ethical imperatives;
- to improve clients' lives;
- it helps us plan effective interventions.

Recent developments in nursing and healthcare in general – for example, the increase in advanced nurse practitioner and nurse consultant roles, as well as the move from hospital to community-based care – have had a dramatic impact on the ways in which nurses practise. The need for an increase in autonomous working while supporting and developing interprofessional and patient-centred approaches to care means that the nurse is required *to always practise in line with the best available evidence* (NMC, 2018b). Such decision-making requires nurses to be familiar with the most current evidence and how this applies to the situations that arise in their practice.

Traditionally, nursing practice was built on an apprenticeship model whereby students learnt to nurse in a manner that reflected what was deemed to represent good nursing by the ward sister and the staff nurses on duty. As such, the way in which nursing care was delivered was based on historical ways of working that had been passed down between generations of nurses with little change and little in the way of questioning (Moule, 2021). Such practices can become ritualised and are practised because 'that is what we have always done'. Not all nursing traditions are bad or detrimental – for example, the traditions of hygiene and cleanliness (first introduced by Florence Nightingale) – at one time more a matter of pleasing matron than anything else – is now known to play a role in infection prevention and control. However, some traditions are at odds with the notions of evidence-based practice that are presented in this book – for example, reusing syringes, because they are undertaken in an unquestioning and unthinking way.

In this section we have identified a number of reasons why evidence-based practice for nursing is essential. We have seen that adopting evidence-informed ways of working is not an optional extra that nurses can ignore if they are too busy. Key among the reasons for adopting a questioning and evidence-based approach to care provision are the ethical arguments about doing good and avoiding harm, the wise use of resources and the development of nursing as a more autonomous profession. In the next section, we will examine what evidence-based practice might actually mean.

Definitions of evidence-based practice

There has been – and there remains – some debate about what evidence-based practice (EBP) actually means. There are many definitions of evidence-based practice, research-informed practice, evidence-based medicine, evidence-based healthcare and evidence-based nursing in the literature. Before we go on to define what we mean by evidence-based practice in this book, and before we explore the concepts that might inform such practice for nursing, it is worth exploring some of these definitions in an attempt to get a feel for what EBP might actually be.

The number and diversity of the definitions demonstrate that there is little agreement between professionals within healthcare as to what exactly evidence-based care means. This can be a source of confusion for student nurses, who should take time to reflect upon what they thought nursing practice was based on before they started nursing, once they started nursing and again as they become more familiar with nursing practice.

Polit and Beck (2020, p2) define evidence-based practice as:

> *the use of the best evidence in making patient care decisions. Such evidence typically comes from research conducted by nurses and other health care professionals.*

This definition places research squarely at the centre of **clinical decision-making** and recognises that such research may come from sources other than just the nursing profession.

Perhaps the most widely quoted definition comes from Sackett et al. (1996, p71), who defined evidence-based medicine as:

> *the conscientious, explicit and judicious use of current best evidence in making decisions about the care of the individual patient. It means integrating individual clinical expertise with the best available external clinical evidence from systematic research.*

This definition identifies a number of important markers of evidence-based practice.

- It is conscientious – it is a purposeful activity one chooses to engage in.
- It is explicit – it is applied in such a way that it can be shown to have been used.
- It is judicious – thought has been given to how it applies to the job in hand.
- It is about the care of the individual patient – the evidence fits the situation one is dealing with.
- It is a mix of individual expertise with knowledge that has been gathered from good quality research.

What Sackett et al. (1996) are saying is that one answer will not fit all clinical scenarios and it is the role of the doctor, in this case, to identify the research that best fits the clinical situation and the patient in front of them. McKibbon (1998, p399) provides a more far-reaching and inclusive definition.

> *Evidence-based practice (EBP) is an approach to health care wherein health professionals use the best evidence possible, i.e. the most appropriate information available, to make clinical decisions for individual patients. EBP values, enhances and builds on clinical expertise, knowledge of disease mechanisms, and pathophysiology. It involves complex and conscientious decision-making based not only on the available evidence but also on patient characteristics, situations, and preferences. It recognizes that health care is individualized and ever changing and involves uncertainties and probabilities. Ultimately EBP is the formalization of the care process that the best clinicians have practised for generations.*

This explanation of EBP goes beyond the other two definitions in recognising the importance of the patient in making decisions ('preferences') about their own care and, as such, perhaps better reflects modern nursing practice incorporating **person-centred care**, which itself is reflected in the national agenda of service user consultation which we identified earlier.

Steglitz et al. (2015) further identify that in the modern healthcare setting, the inter-dependent roles of the various professional groups mean that it is imperative that evidence-based practice models include shared decision-making, which includes the best of the available knowledge from the various professions.

If we are to move the concept of EBP in nursing forward, it is perhaps best to attach it to well-established, patient-focused strategies with which nurses are all familiar. The nursing process of assessing, planning, implementing and evaluating care can be seen to be similar to the stages of implementing EBP that Moule (2021) suggests.

1. Identify a problem from practice and turn it into a specific question.

2. Find the best available evidence that relates to the question, usually by systematically searching the literature.

3. Appraise the evidence.

4. Identify the best evidence alongside the patient's needs and preferences.

5. Evaluate the effect of applying the evidence.

Stage 1 reflects the assessment process in nursing during which the problem to be addressed is identified and framed. Stages 2, 3 and 4 involve a conscientious and explicit planning phase during which the evidence that will underpin the plan is identified and assessed, and the patient's circumstances and preferences are accounted for. This is followed by the implementation of the plan, and the evaluation of the effectiveness of what has been done in the final stage of the nursing process and stage 5 of Moule's (2021) framework.

What is apparent from all these definitions and the application of the nursing process is that EBP is a framework for action and not academic debate and, as such, it places EBP squarely at the heart of nursing practice.

Activity 1.4   Critical Thinking

Thinking about the definitions of EBP, which makes most sense to you? What is it about the definition that makes you think this is the right definition? How will you use the definition to inform the ways in which you work with patients?

As this activity is based on your own observations, there is no outline answer at the end of the chapter.

The approach to the use of EBP is mirrored in the widely cited Critical Appraisal Skills Programme (CASP; see Useful websites at the end of the chapter). CASP asks two important and related questions: How do I know a piece of research has been undertaken properly and that its findings are reliable? When different research points to different answers, how do I know which to believe? The CASP initiative is designed to help care professionals get evidence into practice in three key stages:

1. find the evidence;

2. appraise the evidence;

3. act on the evidence.

This approach mirrors the approach of this book: Chapter 2 tells us how to find evidence from good sources; Chapters 3 and 4 give examples of how to critique research, and Chapters 7 and 8 demonstrate how to put evidence into practice. Find, appraise and act is a good mantra for evidence-based nursing practice. Of course, as with the nursing process, the final stage of the implementation of a plan is to evaluate effectiveness – this is where reflection becomes important for the second time on the EBP cycle (see Chapter 5).

Hierarchies of evidence

This consideration of what evidence-based nursing practice is leads to an important question: if we are to evaluate the research evidence, how do we know which form of research evidence is best and, consequently, what should we do in practice?

Answering the question, 'Which form of research evidence is best?' requires us to do three things. First, we need to understand which forms of evidence might be regarded as suitable for a given question. Second, we need to consider what forms of evidence are the strongest. Third, we need to be able to evaluate individual pieces of research, identifying their strengths and weaknesses, and thereby coming to some conclusion about how good the individual piece of research is. Information on how to address this third step will be covered in more detail in Chapters 3 and 4. Here we will turn our attention to the first and second steps.

As with the definitions of EBP, there is little agreement between different professions and individual practitioners as to what constitutes good evidence; what we do know is that some research approaches (**methodologies**) are better suited to answering certain kinds of questions. This may be surprising to the novice nurse who assumes that everyone knows what they are doing and why they are doing it. In order to understand why there are differences in opinion, it is worth remembering there are many different types of question that arise in nursing practice, and these relate not only to the provision of specific care, but also to how the care is experienced and the relationships between individuals giving and receiving care (see Chapters 3 and 4 for the types of research methodologies that are used to answer specific questions from practice). For now, we should consider what is termed the 'hierarchy of evidence', more often presented as the 'hierarchy of research evidence'.

Hierarchies of evidence give the practitioner and researcher alike some insight into the perceived worth of individual approaches to research. The classic hierarchy of research evidence is given in Table 1.1. It takes account only of **quantitative research** methods and does not allow for **qualitative research** methods or clinical experience or opinion.

Polit and Beck (2020, pii) present a perhaps more useful hierarchy of evidence. This gives some weighting to evidence that takes account of qualitative research as a source of evidence, as well as valuing experience and practice expertise, and other evidence that is not research based (see Table 1.2). This hierarchy is more in line with the concept of evidence that is presented in this book.

	Level	Description
Strongest	1	Meta analyses and systematic reviews – reviews of multiple research reports and the statistics within them.
	2	Randomised controlled trials with definitive results – clinical trials that involve a new intervention that is assessed against another established intervention or no intervention at all and that show a definite result.
	3	Randomised controlled trials with non-definitive results – clinical trials that involve a new intervention which is assessed against another established intervention or no intervention at all, which show a probable result.
	4	Prospective cohort studies/outcomes studies – long-term follow-up studies of large groups of people usually in their natural setting.
	5	Case-control studies – backward-looking studies that demonstrate associations between causes of disease and diseases or other causes and effects.
	6	Cross-sectional studies – studies undertaken in one period in time that measure potential cause and effect simultaneously.
Weakest	7	Case reports – clinical reports of individual episodes of care.

Table 1.1   Example of a classic hierarchy of research evidence

Based on the work of Petticrew and Roberts (2003).

Activity 1.5   Critical thinking

The NMC Standard of Proficiency regarding being an accountable professional requires the nurse to: *use their knowledge and experience to make evidence-based decisions about care* as well as to *understand and apply relevant legal, regulatory and governance requirements, policies, and ethical frameworks* (NMC, 2018a, p8). Do you think that either of the hierarchies of evidence presented in Table 1.1 and Table 1.2 enables you to do this?

There are some possible answers and thoughts at the end of the chapter.

Hierarchies of evidence give the busy nurse some idea about the level of trust they should place in an individual research methodology or review paper. What hierarchies don't do is answer questions about the quality of an individual piece of research (see Chapters 3 and 4), nor do they give any indication of how to deal with an individual patient or clinical question. This is because not all research undertaken using strong research methodologies is itself good quality and because we cannot assume the findings of a piece of research will apply to all patients who are broadly similar to those involved in the research. Hierarchies don't take account of the fact that the question itself is likely to determine the choice of research methodology. Sometimes only one approach will work – for example, it would be pointless attempting to measure survival following surgery using a qualitative method, or studying patient experience using a quantitative one.

	Level	Description
Strongest	1	(a) Systematic review/meta-analysis of randomised controlled trials
	2	Randomised controlled trial
	3	Non-randomised trial
	4	Systematic review of non-experimental studies
	5	Non-experimental (observational) studies
	6	Systematic review/metasynthesis of qualitative studies
	7	Qualitative/descriptive study
Weakest	8	Non-research based – e.g. expert opinion/audit

Table 1.2 Polit and Beck's hierarchy of research evidence

Based on the work of Polit and Beck (2020).

In Chapter 2, ways in which to find and access sources of research evidence are addressed in some detail. It is perhaps sufficient at this stage to have made the point that not all evidence is regarded as equal and that we should be aware that value judgements need to be made when thinking about the types of research evidence we choose to inform our nursing practice. We stated earlier that some questions can only be answered by certain research methodologies, and we should also remember that not all evidence for nursing practice is gained from research; that there are elements of experience and reflection that also need to be accounted for, as we shall see in Chapter 5. We must also be aware that nursing is a person-centred activity and as such the application of evidence must take into account issues of policy, resources, expertise and the individual patient's situation and personal preferences.

On reviewing the hierarchies of evidence you may have noticed that **systematic reviews** appear as the top layer in both examples. Systematic reviews (together with **meta-analyses**) use the data from multiple studies to gain a bigger, and more robust, understanding of a clinical issue. Think of systematic reviews as a means of gathering all the outcomes of similar studies examining similar issues and merging them all together so that the weaknesses associated with any single study become diluted, and the shared strengths of the various studies combine to allow a clear answer to a clinical question to emerge. Systematic reviews include and exclude studies according to very rigid and objective criteria; they assess the quality of the evidence before it is included and provide robust reasons for what they are doing. In this sense, systematic reviews are exactly as described: they are systematic in the application of inclusion and exclusion criteria and in applying criteria to the quality reviewing of existing studies.

Meta-analyses are a way of gathering all the statistical data from various studies and reanalysing it as a whole. As Schmidt and Hunter (2015) indicate, meta-analysis can take studies that are too small to show a statistically meaningful effect individually and combine their data to make useful observations about effect. They suggest that no single study can satisfactorily answer a scientific question on its own.

We do not explain how to undertake or critique a systematic review in this book, but some useful sources of further information are to be found at the end of the chapter. Perhaps the most famous source for accessing systematic clinical reviews is the Cochrane database, which contains in excess of 7,500 reviews of clinical evidence. Systematic reviews should not be confused with simple reviews, as in many review articles. Plain reviews do not necessarily apply any criteria to the search for, nor appraisal of, the literature they include and, in this sense, cannot therefore be said to be *systematic*.

While systematic reviews might sit at the top of the hierarchies of evidence, they do take account of individual circumstances and preferences and so, alongside all of the influences on evidence-based nursing practice, they are a necessary, but not sufficient, individual influence for practice decisions. In the next section of this chapter, we will consider how the various strands of influence might come together in a meaningful way in order to advance nursing practice.

Advancing the meaning of evidence

Typically, the greatest impacts on individual nursing practice are the clinical lessons learnt as students, and indeed, once qualified, the lessons learnt from our nursing and other professional peers. Prior to the explosion of evidence-based practice, the ward sister and the matron dictated the ways in which the nurses worked in their departments and on their wards. This 'sister knows best' working ethos still has a pervasive, and often detrimental, impact on contemporary nursing practice.

What you learn in the classroom, away from practice, often seems remote and unrelated to the realities of high turn-over, stressful nursing practice (Pijl-Zieber et al., 2015). Sometimes lessons learnt appear to be right in the classroom but lose their appeal in the cold light of the practice environment. At other times, it is easier to choose not to discuss or implement such lessons in order to avoid 'rocking the boat' or appearing to be a troublemaker – you might think it is perhaps best to wait until you are in charge to implement what you know to be right. The conflict between what we 'know' and what we do is a source of anxiety for many nurses and student nurses – the anxiety this incongruence between what we know and how circumstances cause us to act is sometimes referred to as **moral distress** (Lamiani et al., 2018).

Activity 1.6   Reflection

Reflect back on a time in practice when the plan of care, and the care delivered to an individual patient made you feel uncomfortable. What was it about the situation that caused you to feel uneasy? What did you do about it at the time? What might you do about such situations in the future? Why?

As this activity is based on your own observations, there is no outline answer at the end of the chapter.

In part, this book lays down a challenge to all nurses, including students, to think about the ethics of what they do and how they do it. It challenges us not only to know what is right, but also to practise in a way that is justifiable.

Clearly, this is a hard thing to ask of any nurse, let alone a student nurse. The question remains, however: if you would want to know the rationale for what someone is doing to you, why would you not provide a rationale for the care that you are providing to someone else? Elsewhere in this series (Ellis, 2020), we make the argument that ethics is everyone's business and that nurses should take responsibility for the choices and the actions they undertake.

This chapter has so far established that EBP is not an exclusively research-driven academic ideal, but more a way of working and questioning (what we refer to as an 'attitude and approach to learning and development' earlier in this chapter) and drawing on sources of knowledge to continuously evolve practice. We have demonstrated that EBP is important for a number of very good reasons and we have come to some conclusions about what EBP is.

It is important at this point to say that there are a number of skills you can learn and attitudes you can adopt in order to develop EBP in your own practice. Unlike most books on evidence-based practice, this book seeks to explore and develop the skills you need to continue to develop as a nurse who practises in an evidence-driven, patient-focused manner. In order to develop these skills, you need to recognise the influences on your thinking and learning, and hence on the way in which you practise. Common influences on how you practise include: what you have been taught in your training; research you have read; experiences you have had; experience of others you have listened to (including those of patients, nurses and other professionals); local and national policies; pressure from managers; and ethical considerations and social norms.

With all these influences on your practice, it is necessary that you consider each situation as a learning experience – that is, that you are willing to learn from and apply learning to each new situation you encounter. As we saw at the start of the chapter, one of the proficiencies the NMC (2018a) require of the registered nurse is that they *demonstrate the knowledge, skills and ability to think critically when applying evidence and drawing on experience to make evidence informed decisions in all situations.* This clearly indicates that learning is not just about believing what you are told or what you read; it is about thinking critically about what you learn and experience, appraising it, considering its usefulness and seeing how it marries up with what you already know (or think you know).

One famous nursing theorist, Carper (1978), identified four ways of 'knowing' in nursing. She labelled these empirical, aesthetic, ethical and personal knowledge (an explanation of each of these is given in Table 1.3). Taken together, Carper suggests that these sources of knowledge give us the 'evidence' on which to base nursing practice.

We have established that there are a number of important influences on the way in which nursing is practised and that there are a range of forms of knowledge that might be used to inform nursing practice. What is needed now is a scheme by which we can draw all these elements together and make sense of not only sources of evidence, but also influences on nursing practice.

Ways of knowing	Meaning
Empirical knowledge	Knowledge found in textbooks or journal papers that is derived from research and that is provable.
Aesthetic knowledge	Subjective and unique knowledge that requires interpretation, creativity, empathy, understanding and valuing. It is knowledge that feels and looks right.
Ethical knowledge	Knowledge based on systems of belief and moral codes of conduct.
Personal knowledge	Knowledge that arises out of experience as sympathy, empathy and understanding.

Table 1.3 Carper's ways of 'knowing' in nursing practice

Based on the work of Carper (1978).

Developing as an evidence-based nurse

In her seminal work, Brechin (2000, p25) presents three pillars for what she calls 'critical practice'; these are presented in Table 1.4. These pillars are tools the nurse can employ to develop an inclusive model of practice, one that recognises the need to want to do what is best for the patient while acting in a manner that respects and includes all the individuals involved, especially the patient, as *The Code* puts it, *to recognise and respect the contribution that people can make to their own health and well-being* (NMC, 2018b). These pillars, or ways of working, require that even as the nurse becomes more practised and knowledgeable in what they do, they take on board and adapt this knowledge in the light of new information, evidence and individual circumstances.

Brechin's pillars tell us something about the sort of person that is needed and the attitude to care that is required of the evidence-based nurse. They support the notions that were advanced earlier in the chapter – that becoming an evidence-based nurse is about making a positive difference and that this difference has to be made in conjunction with their patients and other staff.

Pillar	What this might mean	Example
Forging relationships	Working with others	Being open and honest in communication
Seeking to empower others	Giving back control	Seeking to support patient choices
Making a difference	Improving something	Playing a part in helping someone recover from illness

Table 1.4 Brechin's pillars of critical practice

Based on the work of Brechin (2000).

Many nurse commentators and researchers consider the practice of nursing to be complex (Guarinoni et al., 2015; Olsson et al., 2020). At least some of this complexity derives from the fact that so much of what nurses do is interconnected and not linear or straightforward, so the ways in which we nurse or lead nursing need to reflect this (Cromwell and Boynton, 2020). Complexity might arise in nursing practice when the nurse is required to pay attention not only to the realities of a patient's condition and its treatment (Carper's empirical knowledge), but also to the patient's circumstances and wishes (aesthetic knowledge), the policies and practices of the hospital, their own values and moral codes (ethical knowledge) and their own previous experiences of delivering care to someone in a similar position or with the same disease (personal knowledge).

Leonardsen et al. (2021) identify how one of the key tasks facing practice supervisors is the need to enable them to supervise in the complex environment in which nursing takes place, and to develop the technical and non-technical attributes which allow this to happen. It is the intention of this book to signpost and start to explore some of these attributes and present you, the reader, with options for self-development that will enable you to embrace a life of learning, development and evidenced care-giving.

A model of evidence-based nursing

The model of evidence-based nursing on which this book is based is one of informed nursing action delivered with an understanding and appreciation of the complexity, not only of the information associated with the medical management of a patient, but also of the complex nature of human interaction, beliefs and ethics. Figure 1.1 presents some of the influences on the nurse practising in an evidence-based manner. It shows some of the attributes and skills that need to be developed in order to become an evidence-based nurse and illustrates that all action has to take account of ethical and moral practice.

The rest of the book is given over to examining and explaining these various skills, sources and knowledge. Taken together, they form one proposal for how you might develop to become, and continue to be, an evidence-based nurse.

Activity 1.7   Critical thinking

Adopting the questioning approach to practice (see Figure 1.1), which embraces and juggles many seemingly competing sources of knowledge, while adopting some positive personal attributes or dispositions (characteristics) advocated in Figure 1.1, is seemingly a hard task. There appear to be a large number of things that the nurse needs to do in order to engage with this model. This is certainly true.

(Continued)

Now reflect on your own personal and professional behaviours and orientations to nursing practice. For example, why did you become a nurse and what was it that you thought you might achieve by taking on this role? Which of the attributes do you already possess? Which of these attributes would you like to develop? Can you see any connections between the dispositions? Are there some that you think complement each other?

An outline of what you might find is given at the end of the chapter.

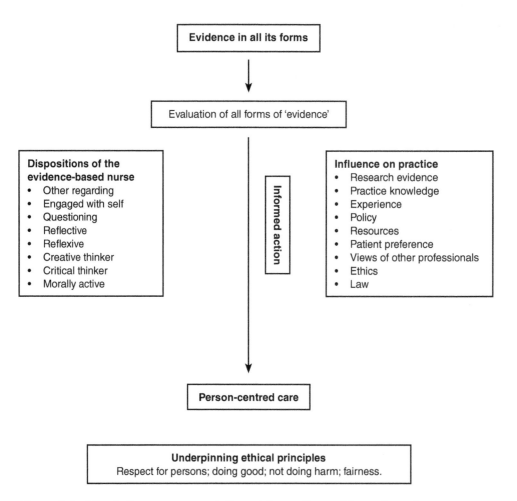

Figure 1.1 The influences on and dispositions of an evidence-based nurse

Chapter summary

This chapter has established that nurses need to identify high-quality sources of knowledge for practice and that they need to critically take account of the quality of the information that these sources present. We have seen that the sources of evidence for practice are not all research based. It has shown that to be a successful evidence-based nurse, one has to engage in lifelong learning and adopt a questioning approach to one's practice. We have also seen that ignoring the evidence base and what we 'know' to be right can be a cause of distress. This chapter has discussed the need to involve the patient and other professionals in decision-making about the patient's care and the fact that research evidence alone does not always provide sufficient grounds on which to base clinical decision-making and action.

Activities: Brief outline answers

Activity 1.2 Reflection (p11)

There is a clear link between our ability as nurses to explain to our patients what we are doing and our ability to explain why we are doing it. All too often nurses are involved in care, but do not understand the rationale behind what they are doing. This will mean that the information passed to patients (in which I include myself and family members) is about what is going to happen and not why or how this will help. Since the 1990s, there has been a growing acceptance among nurses that this is no longer an acceptable way to practise and that as nurses we need to be able to justify what we do in practice to – and, indeed, with – our patients and clients.

Activity 1.5 Critical thinking (p18)

The hierarchies of evidence allow us to make judgements about the likely usefulness of competing forms of evidence in our planning and delivery of care. They suggest quite strongly that some forms of evidence are better than others at informing what we might do and how we do it. Clearly, as with all elements of evidence-based practice, the findings of research need to be interpreted alongside the patient's situation, the skills and resources available, and the patient's preference. We also need to remain cognisant of the fact that even high-quality research methodologies can be poorly applied and therefore individual studies may not be as useful as they might otherwise be. Of course, what these hierarchies miss is that if you want to know what people feel about something – e.g., a medical intervention – then the only useful form of evidence is qualitative and the hierarchy becomes moot.

Activity 1.7 Critical thinking (p23)

What appears clear from the dispositions of the evidence-based nurse is that there are a number of important links between some attributes, such as 'other regarding' and 'morally active'; 'questioning' and 'critical thinker'; and 'engaged with self' and 'reflective'. The development of a more structured approach to questioning, as derived from critical thinking, will also feed into the individual nurse becoming more questioning in general, while adopting a more other focused way of thinking will certainly add something to the nurse's ability to think morally and ethically.

It is probably true that you entered nursing to make a difference to the lives of patients and that you are reading this book because you think it might enhance your ability to do so. This demonstrates that you may already have attributes that include being 'other regarding', questioning and reflective. Learning to see how all of these dispositions come together to create and enhance evidence-based practice is therefore only a matter of consciously engaging with the process of consolidating, developing and exploring the links between attributes that you already have, while being open to cultivating new attributes to complement them.

Further reading

Aveyard, H (2018) *Doing a Literature Review in Health and Social Care: A Practical Guide* (4th edn). Maidenhead: Open University Press.

A clear introductory guide to literature reviewing.

Beauchamp, T and Childress, J (2013) *Principles of Biomedical Ethics* (7th edn). Oxford: Oxford University Press.

This is the most cited ethics textbook covering English-speaking countries and is worth reading to gain an understanding of the four principles of ethics.

Fink, A (2019) *Conducting Research Literature Reviews: From the Internet to Paper* (5th edn). London: Sage.

A more advanced book about literature reviews.

Gerrish, K and Lathlean, J (2015) *The Research Process in Nursing* (7th edn). Oxford: Wiley-Blackwell.

Read Chapter 38 especially. This chapter examines what evidence-based practice might look like.

Moule, P (2020) *Making Sense of Research in Nursing, Health and Social Care* (7th edn). London: Sage.

Read Chapters 1 and 2 especially. These chapters explore the role of research in EBP and also the nature of knowledge for nursing practice in its many forms.

Parahoo, K (2014) *Nursing Research: Principles, Process and Issues* (3rd edn). London: Palgrave Macmillan.

Read Chapters 1 and 2 especially. These chapters explore the role of research in nursing practice and the nature of knowledge for nursing practice.

Polit, DF and Beck, C (2020) *Essentials of Nursing Research: Appraising Evidence for Nursing Practice* (10th edn). London: Lippincott, Williams & Wilkins.

It is worth taking a look at the section about hierarchies and how they relate to the use of evidence.

Useful websites

https://bestpractice.bmj.com/info/benefits-features/evidence-based/

This is an interesting, very clinically orientated website that examines the evidence around a variety of medical conditions and is regularly updated.

https://casp-uk.net

The home of the Critical Appraisal Skills Programme, an Oxford-based organisation concerned with improving the understanding of research evidence in health and social care.

www.cochrane.org

The home of over 7,500 systematic clinical evidence reviews.

www.nice.org.uk/about/what-we-do/evidence-services/journals-and-databases

The website for the National Institute for Health and Care Excellence, which provides access to the latest clinical and non-clinical evidence for practice. This is also a good place to examine some of the criteria NICE uses in order to evaluate medications and interventions for clinical practice.

Chapter 2 Sources of knowledge for evidence-based care

Caroline Thomas

NMC Future nurse: Standards of proficiency for registered nurses (NMC, 2018a)

This chapter will address the following standards of proficiency for registered nurses:

Platform 1: Being an accountable professional

At the point of registration, the registered nurse will be able to:

1.7   demonstrate an understanding of research methods, ethics and governance in order to critically analyse, safely use, share and apply research findings.

1.9   understand the need to base all decisions regarding care and interventions on people's needs and preferences, recognising and addressing any personal and external factors that may unduly influence their decisions.

Platform 2: Promoting health and preventing ill health

2.1   understand and apply the aims and principles of health promotion, protection and improvement and the prevention of ill-health when engaging with people.

Chapter aims

After reading this chapter, you should be able to:

- describe the steps required to undertake a basic online search for evidence;
- identify key sources of appropriate evidence to inform nursing practice;
- demonstrate awareness of sources of health-related policy in the United Kingdom;
- consider the reliability and trustworthiness of some key sources of evidence.

Introduction

Knowing how to search for, access and evaluate information is essential for successful, high-quality, cost-effective practice in professional nursing and healthcare. Acquiring evidence provides nurses with new insights into nursing practice and deepens their understanding of concepts central to nursing care. New insights can also lead to improvements in care. Nurses need to develop a reflective approach to their practice. By finding out about the latest research and evaluating findings, they can use the best available evidence to respond to people's needs. In addition, nurses need to know about the latest policies, standards and guidance determining their practice to ensure their practice is evidence-based. Evidence-based practice requires understanding the process of searching for information and ways of appraising the authority and quality of information sources. The importance of assessing and evaluating sources of evidence is reflected in the Nursing and Midwifery Council (2018a) *Future Nurse: Standards of Proficiency for Registered Nurses.*

This chapter outlines basic search techniques that can be used to find evidence and offers guidance on ways of evaluating the credibility of information found. Defining and refining topics for consideration and following a series of stages to guide research are invaluable in making information searches efficient. This chapter also provides a variety of sources/resources that can be used to access reliable information for evidence-based practice.

To make this chapter relevant to your current requirements, you can search for a topic to assist your assignment writing, or one to deepen your understanding of an aspect of practice. You should bookmark the electronic sources you find or save your searches so that you can return to them in the future.

Scenario

Janice is 26, has completed an access course in health and social care and is starting a pre-registration nursing programme at university. She is anxious to improve her library skills. She finds searching for information challenging and time-consuming. To enhance her ability to research information she undertook a library workshop on 'developing skills for searching for information'.

The workshop content is detailed below.

The search process

Searching for quality information can be time-consuming. Therefore, knowing how to start a search and the steps to follow can ensure effective use of time. Having a search strategy helps prevent you being diverted to information that is connected only loosely to a topic. While you can search manually or electronically, electronic searches can increase the speed and ease of searching. These are emphasised in this chapter.

There are three ways of gaining access to electronically stored evidence: free access, access paid for by institutions and access paid for by individuals. Specialist librarians for nursing, health and social care can provide valuable guidance on what sources of evidence are available and on ways of undertaking searches.

A successful search strategy

A successful search entails collating information about the extent of relevant knowledge available. A straightforward search strategy begins with you defining the topic area and following a series of interrelated steps:

Step 1: Definition of the research question, topic or area of enquiry.

Step 2: Identification of a set of key words.

Step 3: Refining or broadening the search.

Step 4: Identification of appropriate sources of evidence.

Step 5: Keeping a record of the investigation.

Step 1: Defining the research topic or question

Before starting your search, you should determine what you need to find out about and the kind of information required. In practice, this topic may stem from discussions with the people you care for, a review of their notes, or meetings with colleagues or practice supervisors. The subject matter may also relate to a nursing programme's standards or an assessed assignment.

> ### Example: You may wish to find out about the management of high blood pressure.
>
> *A range of factors can contribute to this and there can be a range of treatments, depending on a person's individual needs. Deciding whether you are interested in causes, treatments or both, helps to limit your search and the completion time.*

Step 2: Identification of key words

Identifying key words is essential for successful searches for evidence using indexes in books, electronic databases and search engines, such as Google Scholar. An excellent way to start is to break what you want to find out into a list of key words or concepts. This process can take a few minutes if you are familiar with the topic. Be aware that different wording can be used to describe similar concepts relevant to the topic.

> ## Example: 'Hypertension' means the same thing as 'high blood pressure'.

You can either record the key words in a list or as a mind map. To broaden the list of key words, use of a dictionary or thesaurus can help; however, a general electronic thesaurus may not use a term in the same way as it is used in nursing or medicine.

Another useful source for key words is Wikipedia, a free online encyclopedia. This should not, however, be used to provide references in academic assignments as experts in the field have not necessarily written or reviewed the information. The accuracy of the information can be questioned. *Wikipedia* is covered in the section on appropriate sources of information in this chapter.

Internet search engines, such as Google, Google Scholar or Google Chrome, can reveal a range of items from the search, but not all may be useful sources. By identifying key words, you can reduce the number of hits to a manageable level.

A useful way of identifying key words in a topic is to use the PICO framework (Straus et al., 2010). This can be used to search for studies looking at the outcomes of interventions.

The search question = P + I + C + O

Where:

   P = Problem

   I = Intervention or treatment

   C = Comparison (if needed)

   O = Outcomes.

Useful questions for searches can also be devised using PICO. For example, questions may include:

- *What are the causes of high blood pressure in elderly people?*
- *How can high blood pressure in old people be reduced?*

> ## Example: The following list provides an example of the key words for researching hypertension in elderly people receiving care
>
> - *Blood pressure*
> - *Hypertension*
> - *Old people/patient(s)*
> - *Elderly people/patient(s)*

- *Geriatric(s)*
- *Care*
- *Regulation*
- *Symptoms*
- *Causes*
- *Guidelines*
- *Tests*
- *Risks*
- *Prevention*
- *Signs*

As you start searching, you may be able to expand your list of key words and become more precise in the language used.

Step 3: Refining or extending the search

Once you have a set of words relevant to the search, you can investigate the relationship between the words using electronic sources such as databases, search engines and library catalogues.

Example: 'eating disorders' or 'high blood pressure'

When using Google Scholar as a search engine, a search for 'eating disorders' produces fewer results than a search for eating disorders. The use of inverted commas means that the words will be searched for as a phrase in the order that they are written.

To explore the ways in which two or more key words or search terms relate to each other, you can use *Boolean operators*. These are the link words: AND, OR, NOT. They link key words in a search in a number of ways.

- **AND:** Linking key words with AND narrows a search. You can find sources that contain both key words. You can explore links between specific groups of people with a health condition and symptoms with treatments.

Example: To find out about eating disorders in teenagers, the search would be: teenagers AND 'eating disorders'.

The search will only retrieve items that include all these words. A smaller number of results are found than when just searching for 'eating disorders'.

(Continued)

- **OR:** Using OR broadens a search and allows you to search for several different terms or synonyms used to specify the same thing. Authors may use different terms to describe what you are looking for.

Example: *In looking for evidence on eating disorders in teenagers, OR can be used to describe the same subject: children OR teens OR adolescents OR young adults. Your search could be broadened and include more results by entering: 'eating disorders' AND children OR teenagers.*

- **NOT:** Using NOT narrows a search by excluding unwanted key words. However, be cautious when using NOT to avoid accidental removal of too many results, including relevant results, from the search.

Example: *A search using NOT anorexia excludes information specifically related to this condition. Your search would be: 'eating disorders' NOT anorexia AND teenagers. Alternatively, your search could be: 'eating disorders' AND teenagers NOT anorexia. There will be a slight variation in the number of results found depending on the word order.*

This search reduces the number of hits or results quite significantly.

Another way of refining a search is to set a date or date range on the search. This ensures that the most recent evidence or research is considered. The database may have an *Advanced Search* option. This allows you to specify the date, date range or type of material.

Step 4: Identification of appropriate sources of information

Use authoritative, reliable sources to analyse health-related issues and critically evaluate practice. When tutors mark your assignments, or practice assessors assess your explanation for the care suggested on placement, a key question asked is:

What evidence are you using to convince me that what you suggest/argue is reasonable?

Anecdotal evidence lacks robustness. It is considered unreliable and untrustworthy because it is based on hearsay. Other unsubstantiated forms of evidence also lack reliability and accuracy. There are many sources of information, but those written by people not sufficiently qualified in the field may be inaccurate or flawed. The information may also be poorly written or argued. Use of poor quality, unreliable or anecdotal evidence in a review of evidence or academic assignment can affect the work's credibility. This chapter's section on 'Appropriate sources of information' explores some appropriate sources in depth.

Source of information	Brief description
Experts	Experienced and knowledgeable colleagues, specialists, practice supervisors, patients, carers, social workers.
Libraries and library catalogues	Sources and list of sources held by libraries: university, Trust and NHS evidence libraries.
Journals and e-journals	Peer-reviewed articles and research reports written by different authors. These can be published regularly – e.g., weekly, monthly or annually.
Books and e-books	Textbooks, manuals and electronic books, which generally provide a broad overview of the subject.
News and media	Media-generated health information: newspaper articles, documentaries.
Search engines	Electronic search mechanisms providing access to key organisations, websites and publications.
Key organisations in the field	Publications and websites for National Institute for Health and Care Excellence (NICE), Department of Health and Social Care (DHSC), and Nursing and Midwifery Council (NMC).
Web 2.0 Technologies	A range of websites and applications enable users to create and share content or participate in social networking.
	Examples: Wikis such as *Wikipedia*, blogs, Twitter and Facebook.
Bibliographic databases	Databases providing access to journals, research reports, systematic reviews, conference proceedings, theses.

Table 2.1   The various sources of information available to support professional practice

Authoritative sources recommended by professional staff can be found within university and Trust libraries. When joining a nursing programme, it is important to familiarise yourself with relevant sources of information for use throughout your studies and professional career. Universities may offer workshops or online tutorials and notes on ways of accessing authoritative sources of information. It is important to learn how to use the library catalogue and other electronic databases to access quality sources of information to keep abreast of developments in current practice.

Books, journals and conference papers published by professional organisations related to nursing or scholarly publishers are authoritative texts. Refereed journals are peer reviewed by experts and editors in the field. They consider the quality and credibility of the information. Submissions are required to meet established standards for publication. In contrast, popular periodicals and newspapers can be less reliable sources of information. Still, they can provide helpful overviews of current issues and debates. The reliability of the information depends on the publication.

Policy documents produced by government organisations or professional organisations that improve health and social care are also reliable sources of information.

You may come across a range of views and perspectives on the topics you search for. For evidence-based practice, you should present alternative perspectives, evaluate their usefulness in terms of the question or situation, and present these together with the references to show where you found them.

Systematic reviews can communicate the methods, results and implications of large, complex quantitative studies about a clinical problem undertaken by other researchers. Systematic reviews tend to detail the studies included in the review.

Questions to aid evaluation of the trustworthiness of sources of information

You can ask several questions about various sources of information, particularly web-sites, to check the extent of their reliability and authenticity before you use the information from them. These include the following.

Questions about the author:

- Who is the author of the information?
- Are the author's qualifications and/or professional credentials given to indicate that the author has the authority to write about the field?

Questions about the source/website:

- Who is funding or supporting the website/source?
- Is it an academic website produced by a university or other academic institution, a not-for-profit organisation or a commercial company?
- Who is the intended audience for the website?

Questions about the age of the information:

- When was the information written? The date is often difficult to establish for some websites.
- When was the website created or last updated? Websites are unstable and are continuously updated.
- Is the website and/or the information still relevant?

Questions about objectivity (neutrality) and reliability of content:

- To what extent is the information given objective or unbiased? In being objective, the author should outline limitations of the information or provide a balanced perspective on an issue.
- To what extent does the evidence put forward relate to the claims/arguments being made?
- What is the quality of the writing like?
- Has the information been peer reviewed?
- Does the information fit with what you already know about the subject?

Once you have obtained the evidence, appraise its integrity and applicability to the situation, clinical problem or person to determine whether the findings should be used for academic purposes or to inform practice. If you have doubts about the information, it is best not to use it or to verify it elsewhere from a more reputable source. Such sources could be key organisations for healthcare, specified in the 'Appropriate sources of information' section of this chapter.

Academic websites and key organisations relating to nursing, and bibliographic databases, can provide authoritative, objective information with precise publication dates. You can usually download this in a file such as a PDF. Such sources should ensure that any research studies referred to were approved by an ethics committee and were conducted with the application of ethical principles to protect the interests of research participants.

The way of identifying the type of website accessed

When accessing websites, you can identify the kind of organisation publishing the website and its location using the URL (Uniform Resource Locator). The URL consists of the domain name and several elements – for example, the URL for Google is **www. google.co.uk**.

www   This stands for 'world wide web'.

Google   This represents the sites, which have the rights to use this domain name.

co   This is part of the domain name specifying the type of organisation (co illustrates a corporate organisation/commercial company).

uk   This aspect specifies that it is a UK-based website. However, some websites with .uk may not be located in the UK.

Universities and colleges in the United Kingdom have **ac.uk** at the end of the URL. Local authorities and government organisations have **gov.uk** at the end of the URL, the NHS has **nhs.uk** at the end of the URL. Voluntary, professional, trade union organisations and those acting in the public's interest can have **.org** in the URL. The website for the Nursing and Midwifery Council is an example: **www.nmc.org.uk**. Websites are unstable sources of information. As they are regularly updated and developed, it is essential to reference the date you accessed the information gained.

Step 5: Keeping a record of the search

Please keep a record of the search, the key words used, and when and where they were used. This will enable you to find information again quickly or prevent you from losing track of valuable sources. With electronic searches, you may be able to save your search or print it out. Many bibliographic databases enable searches to be stored for future recall.

When you search online, your search is added to your *search history*. You can view this history following the appropriate onscreen links. You may also be able to edit your search history, save it and print it out so that you can use it again in the future without having to type in the website address or source.

It is possible to save many books and journals found in the electronic library databases. Librarians will be able to advise on this process.

Activity 2.1   Reflection

Janice found the above workshop content helped her to plan and conduct searches. She was also given a list of resources to access when writing her assignments.

Compare the existing ways you have searched for literature with the process described above. How might you narrow down your search for your chosen topic to ensure that it is manageable so that you access the most appropriate literature?

As this activity is based on your own observation, there is no outline answer at the end of the chapter.

Appropriate sources of information

Having established a strategy for organising a search on a relevant topic, you need to consider the usefulness of the information found. Such information may include opinions of experienced practitioners or specialist experts, research-based clinical guidelines and government health policy documents.

Activity 2.2   Research and finding out

Read the varied sources of information available in the remainder of the chapter. Allocate some time to explore the references in the next couple of weeks. Note the type of resource accessed, such as a policy document, practice guidelines or research report. Identify what type of programme assignment or aspect of clinical practice each resource would provide evidence for.

As this activity is based on your own observation, there is no outline answer at the end of the chapter.

Experts

During your nursing career, you will draw on a range of expertise to inform your practice: your personal experience as well as valuable insights or advice gained from the people in your care, carers and colleagues. At the start of your nursing programme, practice supervisors or practice assessors provide considerable guidance, supervision and assessment of your practice. As your programme progresses, you are expected to independently investigate topics in increasing depth, offer an evidence-based rationale for care delivered and question the practice of others. By examining a range of sources of evidence to support practice during your training, you will build up the knowledge and skills base you need throughout your professional career.

Libraries and library catalogues

University libraries

University libraries contain a range of journals and books you can access on the shelves for nursing, which public libraries do not hold. An electronic *library catalogue* provides access to all the library's sources of information. This collection may include e-books, online versions of printed books and electronic journals (e-journals). Consult your programme/module handbook and bibliography for guidance when considering which sources to use.

You can search library catalogues by subject area or author. To locate a book on the shelves, record the class mark (consisting of a series of letters and/or numbers). If the book is out on loan, you may find others with similar class marks on the shelves, covering the topic of interest. You can also search for newspapers, films and large-print books.

Trust libraries

When on placement, you may utilise the Trust's library to aid your academic study and clinical practice. Trust librarians can provide information on your access rights to information, the sources available and ways of utilising the database to conduct searches. As a pre-registration nurse on a university programme, you can apply for free access to NHS Evidence, a library database provided by the National Institute for Health and Care Excellence (NICE). It offers access to a range of e-books, journals and practice guidelines.

Activity 2.3   Critical thinking

Consider the following scenario.

Gillian has started her nursing programme, is confident in her IT and library skills, but was disappointed with her grade in her last academic assignment. The marker's comments suggested that she should make use of more creditable, professional sources of evidence to support her argument and not rely on information from Wikipedia and Google.

What sources of evidence would you recommend that Gillian learns to access?

A possible outline answer can be found at the end of this chapter.

Journal articles

To check the relevance of a journal article identified by a search, read the abstract summarising the article. It usually specifies the kind of information presented. This information can include randomised control trials, systematic reviews and small-scale studies on perspectives of care. The following is a list of some journals particularly relevant to nursing:

- *British Journal of Nursing* (Mark Allen Publishing)
- *International Journal of Nursing Studies (IJNS)*
- *Journal of Advanced Nursing (JAN)*
- *Journal of Clinical Nursing (JCN)*
- *Journal of Nursing Education*
- *Journal of Professional Nursing*
- *Nursing Management*
- *Nursing Practice and Research*
- *Nursing Standard* (Royal College of Nursing, Great Britain)
- *Nursing Times*
- *The Nurse Practitioner.*

By looking at the reference list in relevant articles found you can broaden your search to include other relevant sources of information. It is worth finding out which e-journals for nursing your university library subscribes to.

You need to be aware that some journals have higher academic status than others in the field, as the standards for research reports are more rigorous. These journals tend to be cited more numerously by researchers in the field than others. The *International Journal of Nursing Studies* and *Journal of Advanced Nursing* are highly regarded sources of evidence-based information. The *Nursing Times* is a less rigorous source of evidence-based practice. It publishes professional and clinical news stories and comments from nurses in a 'magazine-style' format.

You may like to ask your health and social care librarian to show how to access the *impact factor* for nursing journals on the Web of Science electronic database. Journals are ranked according to their impact, i.e., the number of times they are cited in other publications and research. Their ranking indicates their academic status in the field of nursing.

Google Books

Searching *Google Books* allows you access to extracts and information from various online books on a topic of your choice. Depending on the viewing rights permitted by publishers, you can obtain a summary of many books, browse the content or index pages, and even read parts or all of the book for free. You can also find out where to purchase or borrow a book you are interested in.

News and media

Newspapers and television provide information on healthcare for the public and up-to-date news items related to issues concerning health and social care provision. By browsing the health pages of newspapers, news programmes and documentaries, you can gain insights into people's perspectives on their care and the findings of reviews of standards of care within Trusts. Articles and news stories can be biased, but the information gathered should stimulate further investigation into the claims made using additional credible sources of evidence rather than being relied upon as the sole justification for altering practice.

Current news items and advice about health can be accessed using websites of some key organisations, news channels and newspapers. Examples include:

- *BBC News*: **www.bbc.co.uk/news/health**
- *The Guardian*: **www.theguardian.com/lifeandstyle/health-and-wellbeing**

Search engines

Many search engines have been designed to help you find information online. These include: *Ask, Bing, Exalead, Google, Google Chrome* and *Google Scholar*. *Google Scholar* focuses specifically on enabling searches for scholarly literature (**https://scholar.google.co.uk**):

From one place, you can search across many disciplines and sources: articles, theses, books, abstracts and court opinions, from academic publishers, professional societies, online repositories, universities and other websites. Google Scholar helps you find relevant work across the world of scholarly research.

Google Scholar offers online advice on searching. It allows you to use key words and Boolean operators covered in this chapter to search for evidence and has an advanced search facility.

Key organisations: websites and publications

You can access a range of reliable, credible evidence from the websites of the key organisations covered in Table 2.2. Understanding the political context governing care in the UK is essential as this impacts upon practice. The Department of Health and Social Care website is one of the most important sources of government policy on health and social care matters in England.

Web 2.0 technologies

Web 2.0 technology makes online communication and collaboration possible. Web 2.0 technologies include social networking and social media sites such as Facebook,

Twitter, LinkedIn, Reddit, Instagram and TikTok. They also include search engines, blogs, wikis such as Wikipedia, apps, podcasts and video-sharing sites such as YouTube. Users can create, share content and comment. For example, users can send text and voice messages or make voice and video calls using the social media app WhatsApp (owned by Meta). Networks, or communities of practice, can be created between similar professionals to share expertise in the field.

Web 2.0 technologies have become a popular means of sharing research findings. They are subject to data protection legislation (Data Protection Act 2018) and the UK General Data Protection Regulation. Social media users can interact, debate aspects of practice and respond to research outcomes.

Blogs can be web-based conversations or diaries around a theme. While contributors' postings may vary in length and quality, blogs illustrate diversity in opinions and comments, concerning news items, policies and health-related issues. In addition, service users can post insightful narratives on their health conditions and care experiences. They may also suggest improvement to practice.

The King's Fund, an independent charity that promotes health and social care in England, has a range of blogs, inviting comment on crucial health and social care issues: www.kingsfund.org.uk/blog. For example, it provides comments on the challenges and opportunities facing health and social care services in response to the Health and Care Act 2022.

Twitter is an online news and social networking site. Users can post and interact with 'tweets'. Politicians capture the **essence** of what they want to say in a limited number of characters to invite interest and engagement. Each 'tweet' has a date for referencing purposes. You can access a range of topics on evidence-based nursing on **https://blogs. bmj.com/ebn/ebn-twitter-journal-club**. The Twitter accounts of key health organisations are listed in Table 2.2.

Caution is needed when using social media sites or blogs in academic work. It is not easy to determine the authority of the information. While the unique perspectives of individuals can be valuable if they are authentic, they can also be biased. Consequently, you should not use the findings to generalise the viewpoints described as being representative of the general population. Gaining insights into a range of perspectives from people receiving care can help you develop sensitivity to the varying needs of patients with specific conditions.

Wikipedia

Wikipedia is a free online encyclopedia and provides a good starting point for finding out about a topic and key words for searches. However, any registered user can alter an article, so it is essential to question the accuracy and authenticity of the information. Articles are continuously being rewritten or updated. References to each entry or topic are often given at the end, and should be checked and compared with other reputable sources.

Key organisation	Website and Twitter accounts	Useful sources of information
Department of Health and Social Care (DHSC)	www.gov.uk/government/organisations/department-of-health-and-social-care **@DHSCgovuk** various social media platforms: Twitter: **https://twitter.com/dhscgovuk** Facebook: **www.facebook.com/DHSCgovuk** Linkedin: **www.linkedin.com/company/dhsc/** YouTube: **www.youtube.com/channel/UCXmtnbNO7_no7RekfUIqVcw**	The DHSC publishes a range of information covering policy announcements, policy consultations and standards relevant to nursing, midwifery and healthcare in the UK. A range of policies, publications on healthcare and national news items related to health can be accessed using the website. Up-to-date statistics on a range of topics such as specific health conditions, births and people's healthcare experiences are also available. There is a link to the NHS for information on its constitution and role. You can access details of the ministers at the DHSC.
National Institute for Health and Care Excellence (NICE)	**www.nice.org.uk** **@NICEcomms** Follow NICE via other social media: Facebook: https://en-gb.facebook.com/**NationalInstituteforHealthandCareExcellence/** YouTube: **www.youtube.com/user/NICEmedia** Instagram: **www.instagram.com/nicecomms/** Linkedin: **www.linkedin.com/company/national-institute-for-health-and-care-excellence/**	NICE is an independent organisation, providing current evidence-based information for health, public health and social care. NICE develops quality standards and guidelines, designed to improve particular areas of health in conjunction with health and social care professionals, their partners and service users. The standards are reviewed annually and can be accessed online. 'Local practice collection', accessible via the website, provides examples of the use of NICE guidance and standards to improve health. The online 'evidence search' allows access to research on a range of topics, links to the Cochrane Library and access to e-books and e-journals using OpenAthens account held with your university library. NICE also provides access to Health Education England's knowledge and library hub resources on evidenced-based practice.

(Continued)

Table 2.2 (Continued)

Key organisation	Website and Twitter accounts	Useful sources of information
NHS England	**www.nhs.uk**	NHS England leads the National Health Service (NHS) in England. It establishes the priorities and direction of the NHS. It encourages and informs the national debate to improve health and care.
Public Health Scotland and Public Health Wales, and	**www.england.nhs.uk** **@NHSEngland** www.healthscotland.com www.nhsinform.scot/	The website provides access to information on people's engagement in healthcare, structure of the healthcare system, the vision for the future and information about health issues.
Health and Social Care Services in Northern Ireland	**@P_H_S_Official** www.wales.nhs.uk/ **@PublicHealthW** http://online.hscni.net **@HSC_NI**	Websites also exist detailing the structure and nature of healthcare provision in Wales, Scotland and Northern Ireland.
Nursing and Midwifery Council (NMC)	**www.nmc.org.uk** **@nmcnews**	The NMC is a statutory body regulating the nursing and midwifery profession to protect the public.

The website provides access to *The Code*: the professional standards of practice and behaviour for nurses, midwives and nursing associates in the UK.

The website provides useful information in the context of care concerning NMC work, projects and priorities. You can access a range of NMC newsletters published regularly, including ones for students, nurses and nursing associates. Each features health and social care developments.

Employers can use the website to check the registration status of employees. |

Key organisation	Website and Twitter accounts	Useful sources of information
Royal College of Nursing (RCN)	www.rcn.org.uk @theRCN	The RCN is a membership organisation for registered nurses, midwives, healthcare assistants and nursing students. As a professional body and trade union, it holds research conferences and campaigns on matters of importance to nurses. It also advises on professional standards, nursing education and nursing practices. The RCN has one of the largest nursing libraries in Europe. Its database enables access to a vast collection of e-books and e-journals. It also produces a range of quality publications. Access to the online version of the *Royal Marsden Manual* provides up-to-date information on nursing skills and procedures. The RCN website provides advice on professional development. A section is devoted to students with resources, events and opportunities to support your studies and search for your first job.
World Health Organization (WHO)	www.who.int (@WHO)	The WHO directs and coordinates international health within the United Nations system. The website provides details of the work of the WHO, its publications, classification of diseases and the tackling of current international health priorities.

Table 2.2 Key health organisations, websites, Twitter or other social media accounts and the information available

Database	URL	Details
Applied Social Science Index and Abstracts ASSIA	https://about.proquest.com/en/products-services/ASSIA-Applied-Social-Sciences-Index-and-Abstracts/	• Provides a comprehensive source of social science and health information for care professionals, academics and students. • Focuses on social problems like addiction and mental illness, covers social and psychological issues and the work of social services. • Contains records from over 500 journals published in 19 countries. • Updated continuously as new content becomes available.
British Nursing Index	https://about.proquest.com/en/products-services/bni	• UK nursing and midwifery database compiled by professional librarians. • Covers over 400 UK journals and other English language titles, including international nursing and midwifery journals, as well as selective content from medical, allied health and management titles. • Typical subjects include medical law, public health and safety, nutrition and psychology.
Cumulative Index to Nursing and Allied Health Literature CINAHL	www.ebsco.com/products/research-databases/cinahl-database	• Provides access to top nursing and allied health literature, including nursing journals, conference proceedings and publications from the National League for Nursing, and the American Nurses' Association. • Literature covers a range of topics such as nursing, biomedicine, health sciences, complementary medicine and consumer health. • Provides access to healthcare books, nursing dissertations, standards of practice, audio-visuals and book chapters.
MEDLINE	https://health.ebsco.com/products/medline	• Created by US National Library of Medicine. • Contains citations and abstracts for biomedical and health journals from around the world. • The Literature Selection Technical Review Committee recommends most of the journals selected. • Used by healthcare professionals, nurses, clinicians and researchers engaged in care, public health and health policy development.
The Cochrane Library	www.cochranelibrary.com	• Produces up-to-date research evidence. • Has several databases. • Cochrane Database of Systematic Reviews (CDSR) is a leading database for healthcare, publishing systematic reviews of randomised controlled trials, editorials and the protocols for Cochrane Reviews. • You can search by topic or each Cochrane Review Group (CGG), which takes responsibility for a specific area of healthcare or policy.

Table 2.3 Examples of subject-specific bibliographic databases relevant to nurses

Bibliographic databases

University libraries subscribe to bibliographic databases. These give nurses access through a username and password to a wealth of published literature, including articles, conference proceedings, research reports, newspaper articles, theses or systematic reviews. Many have menus with on-screen instructions making the retrieval of evidence straightforward. Information is often presented as a reference and a summary of the text. Librarians are able to advise on access rights and use of these.

Full-text resources enable you to download, save and print the full-text version of the article. If you are unable to retrieve the full-text article, make a record of the reference so you can enquire about obtaining this through the library's interlibrary loan system.

Examples of useful subject specific databases

When using bibliographic databases, those relevant to nursing will be most useful to you. These include CINAHL (Cumulative Index to Nursing and Allied Health Literature), British Nursing Index, PsycINFO (which covers aspects related to psychology) and Allied and Complementary Medicine. These all hold references on nursing-related studies. These may be accessible via the internet or your university library.

Activity 2.4   Research and finding out

Select a health-related topic you wish to learn about (e.g., consider the ways of preventing the onset of common colds). Conduct a search using the electronic library catalogue or a search engine of your choice to find three relevant journal articles.

Read the title and abstract for each article. Note the dates of publication. Determine whether they look relevant. Access the full text version and look for information that tells you whether the author is a credible authority on the subject. How detailed is the content? Are references used to support any claims made?

As this is based on your own observation, there is no outline answer at the end of the chapter.

Chapter summary

This chapter has outlined the following:

- Appropriate sources from within and outside the nursing field to assist evidence-based practice.
- The importance of planning a search strategy, making notes and following a simple process for conducting searches for evidence using key words and Boolean operators.

(Continued)

- Questions that you can use to help evaluate the quality and authority of sources of evidence.
- The need to familiarise yourself with sources of information that are most relevant so that these can be revisited regularly to help you keep up to date with developments in practice.
- The importance of seeking support from subject specialist librarians on sources of information and searches.

The better informed you are as a nurse, the more likely you are to provide high standards of care and achieve successful outcomes for the recipients. This chapter has encouraged you to seek out the information you need to provide good care for people and prepare for your written assessments.

Activity: Brief outline answer

Activity 2.3 Critical thinking (page 37)

Gillian may find it helpful to use Google Scholar to access more academic material to use in her assignments. She could also enquire about tutorials or workshops to assist her in the use of the library catalogue.

She will need to master ways of accessing bibliographic databases so that she can access full-text journal articles.

She could access more professional sources of information through using websites such as NICE, NMC and the Royal College of Nursing. Websites such as the Department of Health and Social Care will help her develop an understanding of the influence of policy on practice.

Further reading

Gerrish, K and Lathlean, J (eds) (2015) *The Research Process in Nursing* (7th edn). Chichester: John Wiley & Sons.

Moule, P, Aveyard, H and Goodman, M (2016) *Nursing Research: An Introduction* (3rd edn). London: Sage.

Nursing and Midwifery Council (2018) *Future Nurse: Standards of Proficiency for Registered Nurses.* Available at:

www.nmc.org.uk/globalassets/sitedocuments/standards-of-proficiency/nurses/future-nurse-proficiencies.pdf

Schmidt, NA and Brown, JM (eds) (2021) *Evidence-based Practice for Nurses: Appraisal and Application* (5th edn). Burlington, VT: Jones & Bartlett.

Useful websites and Twitter accounts

www.bnf.org/

British National Formulary (BNF) publications provide doctors, pharmacists and other healthcare professionals with sound, up-to-date and timely information on drug selection, prescribing, dispensing and administration.

www.cqc.org.uk

@CareQualityComm

The Care Quality Commission (CQC) website for the independent regulator of health and social care in England enables access and comparison of service ratings for care services, such as care homes and hospitals. It also provides access to commissioned research reports and inspection reports for care services.

www.england.nhs.uk/about/equality/equality-hub/resources/evidence/

@NHSEngland

National Health Service provides access to a range of evidence, including the health profiles of local authorities, social determinants of health and quality of health services.

www.gov.uk/government/organisations/department-of-health-and-social-care

@DHSCgovuk

Department of Health and Social Care website provides access to national health policy information.

www.kingsfund.org.uk/topics/public-health

The King's Fund is an independent charitable organisation working to improve health and care in England. Its website provides access to blogs and independent research on health and social care.

www.ons.gov.uk

@ONS

The Office for National Statistics website provides statistical data on diseases and treatments that can be used to explain the context of a health topic. An example includes the mortality rates for heart disease and cancer.

Chapter 3 Critiquing research: general points

Peter Ellis

Chapter aims

After reading this chapter, you will be able to:

- demonstrate awareness of the need for critical appraisal of research in health and social care;
- describe the type of questions that can be applied to all research papers during the critiquing process;
- demonstrate awareness of the systematic nature of the process of research critiquing;
- understand the ethical considerations that need to be taken into account when evaluating health and social care research.

Introduction

In this book we have established that it is important for nurses who wish to be truly evidence-based to be critical and analytical in their approach to the identification, reading and potential adoption into their practice of various sources of evidence. We have already indicated that an understanding of research methodologies, **methods** and analysis is useful in establishing the worth of **empirical** literature to inform evidence-based nursing practice.

The opportunities for every nurse to engage in clinical research are limited, and there are good reasons why this should be the case. Prime among these is the potential for overwhelming both practice and patients with requests to participate in research, thereby detracting from the delivery of good quality clinical care. Rather, the challenge is for nurses to engage with research as an important source of evidence to guide and inform practice. One practical mechanism for doing this is via a work-based or university journal club that might meet to identify, critique and discuss the adoption of new research findings.

Renewal of registration and revalidation according to *The Code* Paragraph 22.3 (NMC, 2018b) requires nurses to *keep your knowledge and skills up to date, taking part in appropriate and regular learning and professional development activities that aim to maintain and develop your competence and improve your performance.* Clearly, one of the requirements for revalidation of nurses is that they engage in continuing professional development and that they maintain a record of reflection; it would therefore be a good habit for nursing students to develop and registered nurses to continue with (Ellis and Abbott, 2015).

Regardless of whether all nurses are able to undertake research, they should have at least a basic understanding of how research is undertaken and what constitutes good-quality research fit to inform their practice. Being able to judge the quality of a piece of research and its applicability to our individual clinical settings and client groups is essential if we are to use it to inform what we do in a meaningful way. So as well as being able to critique research, nurses need to understand whether the research might be useful in informing practice where they work and with the people they work with. As we have seen above, one of the proficiencies expected of the registered nurse by the NMC (2018a) is that they *demonstrate an understanding of research methods, ethics and governance in order to critically analyse, safely use, share and apply research findings to promote and inform best nursing practice.* The important bit of this proficiency for this chapter is that you learn to critically analyse research in order that you can apply it, along with the other forms of evidence identified in Chapter 1, to your practice as a nurse.

It is beyond the scope of this book to look in detail at the design and execution of the various forms of research used to inform nursing practice. For a detailed look at the design and undertaking of research studies in nursing practice, or to help you with a critique of a piece of research, see *Understanding Research for Nursing Students* (also in this series – other sources you may wish to use are identified at the end of this chapter).

Because there is a need to understand some general areas for critique, as well as how to critique the specifics of the two main research **paradigms**, qualitative and quantitative, and their methodologies, this part of the book is split into two chapters. This chapter, the generic section, deals with critiquing elements of published research that apply to *all* research papers of whatever methodology. This includes the titles, authors, choice of research paradigm, and the discussion and conclusions sections of the paper, as well as some consideration of the ethical questions that might be asked of a published study. The next chapter (Chapter 4) will focus on specific questions to be asked of qualitative and quantitative research. Areas for critique within Chapter 4 include methodological choice (design), sampling, data-collection methods, the quality of the research process and analysis of the data.

Within both chapters there are some brief descriptions and critiques of elements of various research papers. Most of these papers are readily available via university or hospital-based journal subscriptions, both online and on paper. Where possible, it would help your understanding of the process of research critiquing to read some of these papers in full, although this is not absolutely necessary. Chapter 2 has already shown you how to work out how to access these papers using electronic database searches – the details of which are explored in *Information Skills for Nursing Students*, also in this series.

As well as the guidance contained within these chapters there is a comprehensive critiquing framework in the Appendix that can be applied to most research. This framework is in three sections: the first applies to all research, as does this chapter; the second has additional questions that apply to qualitative research (see Chapter 4); and the third has additional questions that relate to quantitative research (also in Chapter 4). You might find it useful to read both chapters while simultaneously referring to the questions contained in this framework. Because the critiquing of research is a dynamic process where a number of judgement calls need to be made, the contents of the chapters and the questions within the framework do not exactly mirror each other.

It is important to establish right from the start that critiquing in this sense is seen not merely as an activity that is used to identify weaknesses within a study, but also as an activity that seeks to establish a study's strengths and therefore the degree of faith that can be placed in its findings. So, as in the rest of the book, the critical activities are seen not merely as a means to establish weakness, but also as a means of identifying good-quality evidence that may subsequently be useful in the advancement of practice. Clearly, this cannot be achieved if the sole intention of the activity is to identify and discard weak research.

The format of the presentation of this and the following chapter is intended not only to help you ask the right questions of the different areas of the research papers you read, but also to provide you with what you might be looking for in the way of a positive answer to the questions posed. The questions and guidance in these two chapters, along with the framework in the Appendix, can be used to provide a map for undertaking a critique of a research paper in a meaningful and straightforward manner.

While much of what you will need to ask and the sorts of answers that you will be looking for is contained within these chapters and the Appendix, this does not negate the need for some further reading around the methodologies and methods of the papers you may be using these chapters for to help you critically analyse.

If you are undertaking a critique as part of some coursework, you should also refer to the assignment guidelines and ensure that you only appraise the elements of the research you are asked to critique. Very often the guidelines will identify a particular critiquing framework to use; if not, then you might choose to use the one in this book or one of the many methodology specific checklists that are on the Critical Appraisal Skills Programme or Joanna Briggs Institute websites identified under Useful websites at the end of the chapter, or within a number of research and evidence-based practice textbooks and journal papers also identified at the end of the chapter.

Undertaking the critique

There is no single right way to approach undertaking a critique of a piece of research. There are, however, some strategies that will make the process easier for the novice to undertake and that can provide structure to the process.

Lobiondo-Wood and Haber (2013) suggest the following strategy:

- Skim read the paper to get a feel for the overall approach of the research.
- Read the paper in depth, making sure you understand each element.
- Break the study down into its component parts.
- Think about the study as a whole and consider its message.

These are useful strategies that are helpful not only to novice readers of research, but also to those who have more experience of reviewing and critiquing research. Highlighting important areas of the text is also useful, as is drawing a simple flow diagram of the research, including the research question/aims, methodology, sample, methods, analysis, results and key discussion points, which makes referring back to the paper much easier to do and aids in the critiquing process (see Figure 3.1). A short overview of each piece of research is very helpful where you are considering critiquing a number of research papers, as you might in a review or when writing an essay using several pieces of research, for example.

A much briefer flow diagram of such research can prove useful for gaining an overview of a single piece of research and for comparing the processes with a number of different research studies. In fact, the Consolidated Standards of Reporting Trials (CONSORT) group, who are concerned with improving the reporting of clinical trials, have created a flow diagram for this very purpose, which demonstrates how data can be downsized into manageable chunks for the purposes of review. Clearly, this template applies only to clinical trials and shows participant movement through a trial, but the idea can be adapted to suit all research methodologies and further notes can be added as required.

Activity 3.1 Research and finding out

Visit the CONSORT website at **www.consort-statement.org/consort-statement/flow-diagram** and download a copy of the diagram. Take some time to look over the way in which it is presented, and consider how you might use and adapt it for yourself. If you are undertaking a critique or collecting research reports as part of your coursework, consider using this flow diagram to help structure what you do.

As this activity is based on your own observations, there is no outline answer at the end of the chapter.

Furze, G, Cox, H, Morton, V, Chuang, L-H, Lewin, RJP, Nelson, P, Carty, R, Norris, H, Patel, N and Elton, P (2012) Randomized controlled trial of a lay-facilitated angina management programme. *Journal of Advanced Nursing*, 68 (10): 2267–79.

↓

Aims: To establish the relative effectiveness and comparative costs associated with a home-based, lay-facilitated angina management programme when compared to routine advice and education from a a specialist nurse.

↓

Methodology: Randomized controlled trial.

↓

Sample: Adult patients with angina in rapid-access chest pain clinic at a district general hospital; excluding: need for urgent revascularisation, exercise-induced arrhythmias, loss of systolic BP greater than 20mmHg during exercise stress testing, increasing number and duration of attacks of angina; a score of 4 on the Canadian Angina Class or the New York Heart Association classification of heart failure; life-threatening co-morbidities; certain psychiatric problems. 142 recruited (sample size calculation suggests 158).

↓

Methods: Intervention group: Angina Plan (education about angina, exercise, stress management referrral for smoking cessation) delivered and monitored by trained lay persons. Control group: seen by specialist nurse in clinic and given usual advice.

↓

Analysis: Intention to treat analysis (includes withdrawals to reflect true life). Regression modelling used, number of angina episodes over six months plus blood pressure, cholestrol, body mass index, waist/hip ratio, Seattle Angina Questionnaire and Hospital Anxiety and Depression Scales. Cost-effectiveness assessed using Quality Adjusted Life Years.

↓

Results: No important difference in frequency of angina at six months. Positive differences for intervention group, at three months for anxiety, understanding and exercise; and at six months for anxiety, depression and understanding. The intevention was considered cost-effective.

↓

Discussion: Some outcomes are better within the Angina Plan delivered by lay persons than standard advice presented in the clinic by a specialist nurse.

Figure 3.1 Example overview of a randomised controlled trial

A further useful (and often overlooked) part of the process of an academic critique is the use of research resources to inform the process. This involves using books about research to highlight the processes a research study might undertake in the ideal world. What actually happened in the study you are reviewing is then compared to these processes as part of your critique. Of course, it is often the case that you will understand different sections in certain books better than in others, so use more than one textbook against which to compare the research that you are reading. Some useful textbooks and journal papers are listed in the Further reading at the end of the chapter.

Theory

When undertaking an assignment as part of a course or module of study, it is usual to follow certain academic conventions. The need to follow these conventions is no different when undertaking a critique. The usual strategy when approaching this sort of work is to define your terms (explain what a technical word means), reference the definition (to an academic text such as a research textbook), and apply the definition to the critique you are undertaking. There is then a higher probability that you understand the new terminology and that the marker understands what it is you are trying to say and is sure that you understand what it is you are saying; this process of define, reference and apply is a good tool for all forms of academic work.

Many textbooks and websites about research and evidence-based practice contain frameworks that can be used to guide the process of critiquing a research paper (see the Further reading section at the end of the chapter). They point the reader in the direction of the correct questions to ask at the different stages of the review; in general, they are best used in conjunction with at least one research textbook. It is important to ascertain what types of research the frameworks are written in relation to, as some are generic (that is, they apply to all methodologies), while others are specific to either the **qualitative** or **quantitative paradigms**, and yet others relate only to individual specific methodologies. The critiquing framework presented in the Appendix is both generic (it can be used to ask questions of all research methodologies) and specific (it contains paradigm-specific elements).

Concept summary: quantitative and qualitative research

Quantitative research is associated with scientific enquiry that views the world in a measurable, 'provable' manner. 'Quantitative' refers to the fact that findings are countable or can be presented in numbers, tables and graphs. Quantitative research is concerned with proof, with cause and effect, and with demonstrating associations. Quantitative research often starts with a **hypothesis**, an idea to be tested using scientific methods.

Qualitative research is associated with the social sciences and 'people-centred' enquiry. 'Qualitative' refers to looking at the world from the point of view of what people feel, think,

(Continued)

understand and believe – things that cannot easily be measured or counted. It is not so concerned with proof as with describing and understanding experiences from the viewpoint of people who have had, or are having, the experience in question. Qualitative research starts with a question and may be used to generate a hypothesis, but does not start with one.

General questions

There are some questions that apply to all the research papers you might read. These general questions relate to some of the core decisions about the overall approach to the research being undertaken, how ethically the research has been undertaken and, to a lesser extent, the title of the paper and the credentials of the authors. Some common pitfalls and assumptions that students make when critiquing research will be identified below, along with some ideas about how to overcome these and establish the quality of the critique being undertaken.

This notion of the quality of the critique is in many respects as important as the notion of the quality of the research paper. If the idea of learning to prepare, and indeed to undertake, a research critique is to provide evidence to inform clinical practice, then the process by which this is achieved must also be robust. Clearly, this is also important for the student who is seeking to gain a good mark for a piece of course work as well!

Title

Many critiquing frameworks require the user to make decisions about the quality of some issues relating to the title of the paper being critiqued. Certainly, it is very frustrating to find that the content of a paper bears no resemblance to what appears in the title. There can also be an issue with being able to identify from a paper's title that it is a research paper rather than a review or an opinion piece.

The truth of the matter is that more often than not the authors of journal papers have limited input into the title their paper is given. The journal staff sometimes choose the title of the paper as a means of attracting potential readers to both the individual article and the journal.

Activity 3.2   Critical thinking

When reading a journal paper, what are the clues that it is original research rather than a review or opinion paper? List some of the features that are different between research and other forms of paper.

An outline answer is provided at the end of the chapter.

If you are required to critique elements of a research paper such as the title as part of some coursework, then you must; ordinarily, however, it is not considered an important element of the critiquing process. As a general rule, a good title will identify the characteristics of the participants (e.g., people with diabetes), the nature of the research questions (e.g., quality of life) and the methodological approach used (e.g., **phenomenology**). Some titles may also include some message about the key findings of the research, although this is not always possible. A bad title does not mean that the research itself is bad (Coughlan and Cronin, 2017).

Author credentials

In essence, the author credentials are not as important as the quality of the research itself, as all researchers have to start with a first paper and therefore limited publishing credentials (Coughlan et al., 2007). Checking the authors' credentials requires understanding of at least one of three main areas: their qualifications, their current and past work roles, and their publication history.

It may be preferable for someone undertaking nursing research to have a nursing background, and this may be established within the paper. Many journals do not publish authors' qualifications, however, so this is not always easily ascertained. It would therefore not be possible to critique credibility from this angle.

The author's role(s) can give a reasonable insight into what experience they have of the topic at hand – many journals publish this. Although we said that it may be preferable for nursing research to be undertaken by nurses, this certainly does not exclude research undertaken by people with other professional or academic backgrounds. Much of the knowledge base for nursing has been gained from other professional and academic disciplines, so it is common for individuals other than nurses to contribute to or undertake research that is applicable to nursing.

The third strategy that can be applied to establishing the author's credentials is to look at their publication history. This can often be achieved by finding their profile(s) (where these exist) – for example, on a university website – and where these are not available, by doing an author search on a bibliographic database to identify papers they have published on the topic of interest. A note of caution: sometimes the author with the research expertise is not the first author – for example, when a lecturer publishes work together with a research student, it may be necessary to search for more than just the first author. Again, just because someone is publishing research for the first time does not mean the research is not of a good quality.

Activity 3.3 Research and finding out

Go online and search out the profiles of one or more of the lecturers or professors at your university. See if you can discover what qualifications they have, what their research interests are, as well as what publications they might have. Consider what that means for their credibility in relation to what they teach at the university.

As this activity is based on your own observations, there is no outline answer at the end of the chapter.

The choice of research paradigm

The choice of research paradigm will depend on the type of question, or questions, that a piece of research is setting out to answer (Polit and Beck, 2020). Essentially, in health and social care (including nursing) research there are two distinct research paradigms. These paradigms represent two distinct, but not entirely separate, philosophical ways of viewing the world and asking questions. You may be familiar with the terms for these philosophical approaches: the qualitative paradigm and the quantitative paradigm (see Concept summary on p53).

Given the differences between quantitative and qualitative paradigms, it is apparent that the approach to answering a question arising from nursing practice will depend on the nature of the question being asked. Questions that focus on how people experience their world, what their attitudes are and how they perceive things will sit within the qualitative paradigm, and will require that qualitative methodologies and methods are used to investigate them, while questions about cause and effect and things that can be counted will require quantitative methodologies and methods. The two world views are not interchangeable in terms of asking specific research questions; however, many authors use methods for research data-collection that are questionable, given the question they are posing. For example, it is quite common to see questionnaires used to collect qualitative data, but, as we shall see, the value of questionnaires (essentially a quantitative method) in qualitative research is itself questionable. The wrong choice of research methodology will always mean that the research aims and objectives cannot be met, because the research is fatally flawed.

Concept summary: triangulation

Given the differences in approach to asking and answering questions, it would seem logical to expect to see research using either a qualitative or a quantitative approach to answering questions. While this is often the case, some research employs mixed methodologies and methods in order to look at a research question from more than one angle – this is called **triangulation**.

This triangulation of methodologies and methods allows the researchers not only to ask questions about *what* happens under which circumstances and *how* it happens (as in quantitative research), but also to explore *why* people behave as they do or have the beliefs and opinions that they express (as in qualitative research). For example, *quantitatively* it can be demonstrated that a diet that is high in saturated fats is bad for health. In order to address individuals' eating behaviours, however, it is first necessary to understand, using *qualitative* methods, why people make the lifestyle choices they do.

The background/introduction/literature review, which is at the start of all good research papers, will help establish the credentials of the study as a qualitative or quantitative study (Moule, 2021). A good introduction will explore the state of the literature about the topic of interest and will establish what important older (but recent where possible) research has shown about it.

Essentially, it is usual for the argument put forward in the introduction to the paper to lead the reader to the point where they can appreciate the sorts of questions that need answering about the topic of the research.

It is these questions posed in the introduction that will frame the research as either quantitative or qualitative.

Example critique: choice of paradigm

Humphreys et al. (2021) used a qualitative research methodology in their study of the lived experience of people with long COVID focusing on their levels of physical activity. Since this study is concerned with the experiences of the participants and not measuring medication use or hospitalisation, for example, then a qualitative methodology is wholly appropriate.

Questions posed in quantitative research are about counting, proof, about cause and effect, and demonstrating potential associations between **variables**. Quantitative research often starts with a hypothesis, which is essentially an idea that is tested using established scientific methods. Hypotheses are often presented as a **null hypothesis** (or the opposite of what the researcher actually expects to find) in order to aid statistical analysis, which will disprove the null hypothesis, or prove the hypothesis, if you like.

Example of a quantitative research hypothesis

In their study to evaluate the effectiveness of a nurse-supported self-management programme to improve social participation in older adults with dual sensory impairment, Roets-Merken et al. (2018) posed the hypothesis that the self-management programme for individuals with dual sensory impairment would positively affect their social participation. Since this is an interventional study and quantitative tools can be used to enumerate participation in self-management and quantify social participation, this appears to be a reasonable hypothesis which it is possible to test.

Qualitative questions seek answers about things that cannot easily be measured, counted or proven. They are more concerned with understanding experiences, opinions and beliefs. Qualitative research starts with a question, an aim, an objective or a general statement about something that needs exploring; it does not start with a hypothesis, but may be used to generate one. That said, it is important that the aim or objective of qualitative research is clearly discernible so that the researchers, and subsequently the reader, can see that the research has achieved what it set out to achieve, even if this is just to explore a general topic area.

Example of a qualitative research objective

In their qualitative study to understand the experiences of people living with Parkinson's disease, Merritt et al. (2018) pose the objective of their study as being to describe the experience of being diagnosed and living with mild to moderate Parkinson's disease. Given that qualitative research is **inductive**, this objective, which contains no reference to the findings of the study and does not pose a hypothesis, appears to be appropriate to this research enquiry.

Critiquing the choice of paradigm, therefore, requires that you know what the two research paradigms are used to investigate and the sorts of questions they can answer. On some occasions it appears evident from the introduction that the answers to the important questions being asked lie in more than one paradigm, and the researcher may be under-investigating the topic by failing to use a triangulated methodology.

Ethics

Ethics should permeate the whole research process. Good research is ethical research, but sadly not all ethical research is good research. Certainly, it is possible to undertake research that is both ethical and of a high standard, and in many respects producing research ethically adds to the quality of the research process, especially where it has been subject to the review process.

When critiquing research from an ethical point of view, there are many questions that can and should be asked. Many students look for some statement that the research has been given ethical clearance, and many regard this as showing that the research is therefore ethically sound. There are two problems with adopting this stance: the first is that not all papers make this statement (Jolley, 2020); and the second is that, even with ethical clearance, there may still be questions about the conduct of the research that need to be answered.

Concept summary: critiquing journal papers

One note of caution for the novice at critiquing is that many journals only accept papers that can demonstrate ethical clearance at the point of submission. In such journals, the individual papers will not state that they received ethical clearance. It is worth checking either inside the journal itself or on the journal website where they carry 'information for authors' for a statement about the requirements for demonstrating ethical clearance for all research papers prior to acceptance – not only will this inform your critique, but it is likely to impress your marker too.

Critiquing the ethical credentials of a paper starts with asking questions about whether the research was necessary or whether the existing research, which is covered in the introduction and literature review at the start of the paper, suggests it is not. Undertaking research that is unnecessary is ethically questionable because of the use of resources, including people's time and energy. One also has to consider the emotional investment that people make in the research process where they hope that the research they are participating in may be of benefit to them or to other people in the future; it is therefore unethical to ask people to participate in research that has previously been proven to be futile or of general benefit; in the latter case, people should just be offered the **gold standard** care.

Gaining **consent** is an ethical cornerstone of any research. Gaining true and valid consent is especially challenging in health and social care research because the participants have the potential to be vulnerable. This vulnerability may result from the participants being ill, elderly or in a dependent relationship with the researcher (who may also be their nurse or otherwise involved in their care). Gaining true consent requires the researcher to demonstrate that the participants' agreement to participate has been free from any coercion, either real or potential (Beauchamp and Childress, 2013).

Coupled with the issue of potential coercion are questions about the ability of the individuals to make a choice about whether to take part in a study or not. This freedom of choice is best illustrated in those studies that report that the participants know that they do not have to take part in the study and that they are aware that they can withdraw at any stage without compromising their usual care – although where this is not stated, it is hard to know if this principle has been observed.

Consent also requires that the potential participants have the **capacity** (mental ability) to make the choice to participate or not (Ellis, 2020). If there is any doubt about capacity, it is desirable that other sources of consent are sought – for instance, from spouses, parents or other guardians (this is sometimes referred to as **assent**). In studies where there are obvious questions about the capacity of the participants to consent to taking part, it is desirable that the researchers make some statement about ethically managing this.

Example critique: consent

In their study into perceived issues with eating and drinking difficulties in people living with dementia, Anantapong et al. (2021) only included people in the study if they had enough mental capacity to be able to provide 'informed consent'. This demonstrates that Anantapong et al. are showing respect for persons by not exploiting people who are incapable of providing consent, although given that the main method used for data collection was semi-structured interviews, there are also practical reasons as to why the participants with dementia need the capability to communicate.

Other fundamental questions to be asked of the ethics of a paper include: Do they protect the **confidentiality** and **anonymity** of those involved? Do they appear to have done more good than harm? Did the study answer the question as set and were the resources used in the study used to good effect?

Activity 3.4   Reflection

Review what *The Code* says about consent and confidentiality. Reflect on what this means for undertaking nursing research.

As this activity is based on your own reflection, there is no outline answer at the end of the chapter.

All of these ethical questions can be asked in the critique, especially where the paper does not explicitly state whether the researchers have addressed them. A good study will not only state what ethical questions there are, but also suggest how these might have been addressed. For example, a good paper will make it clear that the researchers dealt with any upset caused by making counselling and support available.

There are many sources of questions about the ethics of research and how these should apply to the conduct of research in human subjects. Some general ethical principles that guide this questioning have already been identified, but Beauchamp and Childress (2013) identify four important ethical principles that apply to all healthcare practice and might inform a critique. These principles were introduced in Chapter 1 and are: **beneficence** (doing good); **non-maleficence** (avoiding unnecessary harm); **autonomy** (respecting freedom of action) and **justice** (fairness).

Critiquing the ethics of a piece of research is as much about your understanding of what is right, what is wrong and what might be ethically questionable as it is about following a critiquing framework. This is one reason why having an understanding of *The Code* is important and why you were asked to review it in this chapter.

The discussion and conclusions

The purpose of the discussion and conclusions sections of the paper is to add some context to the results section. Context is achieved by reviewing how well the research has answered the initial question asked (or demonstrated the hypothesis to be true) or not, as well as examining what similar research in the same area has shown and perhaps looking at the policy context within which the findings might operate (Gerrish and Lathlean, 2015).

The discussion also allows the researcher to explain the results that they have found and why they may have arrived at them. The discussion section of a research paper may be presented in one of two ways: it may be a section on its own or it may be contained within the results section with a discussion attached to each of the results. Either style is reasonable.

From the critiquing point of view, there are two common problems that arise in the discussion sections of published research. First, they may be used to expand on the results rather than explain and contextualise them, and second, the discussion of the results may wander away from a discussion of the questions that were originally posed. This final point can be devastating for a paper that has failed to actually address the question it set out to answer. This wandering of the discussion often points to the use of the wrong methodology or data-collection methods, or to the fact that the authors have been distracted from their main aim by incidental, albeit exciting, findings.

Incidental findings that were not part of the original aim of the research can be of questionable value, as the research design, methodology and methods were not chosen to enable the researchers to answer the incidental question – that is to say, the incidental findings may be subject to **biases**, or other issues with quality, that the researcher has not anticipated that may mean the findings are of questionable worth.

Theory

By creating a flow diagram of the contents of a research paper, it is easy to identify the initial question or hypothesis that the research set out to answer. This can then be used to compare the results identified in the discussion with the initial aims of the study to see if the two are consistent. Not only does this save time, but it adds to the clarity of the process (see Figure 3.1).

The discussion section of the paper is also the place where researchers can discuss the limitations of the study that may arise from practical issues with the implementation of research or from issues that were not fully thought out at the start of the study process. Identifying the methodological and other weaknesses of a study in the discussion and conclusions allows the reader to appreciate some of the tensions that present themselves when trying to do research in the real world. The fact that the author identifies issues with the design or implementation of the research should lead them to be a little circumspect over the findings/applicability of their paper; where this is not the case, it is certainly worth a mention in the critique.

The best conclusions relate only to the aims of the study and what other research and policy might mean in relation to the findings. It is the nature of nursing and all health and social care research that the findings from a study generate new questions that need answering.

Such questions may arise out of the findings of the research, the lack of definitive findings from the research, or perhaps contradictions between the study and other previous research or existing policy. The diligent researcher will recognise these issues and will suggest areas for further research, which may be presented as questions or general topic areas. Where a paper lacks suggestions for further research, it tends to suggest that the researchers have failed to understand the contribution of their paper to the wider understanding of the topic being investigated; the novice nurse might not know what questions should arise following a study, but they can comment when they are not there.

Chapter summary

This chapter has introduced you to the key elements that need to be considered when setting out to undertake a critique of a piece of research and has established why it is important to be able to critique research before considering applying its findings to nursing practice.

There are many methods available to the novice – and, indeed, to the experienced nurse – that help in the process of appraising a piece of research. These include creating an overview and/or flow diagram of the research to highlight important areas and using a critiquing framework supplemented with research methodology textbooks and journal papers to guide the process.

A variety of issues must be considered when critiquing the title of a research paper, including the credentials of the researchers undertaking the study. Sometimes a degree of detective work is necessary in order to critique these in a meaningful way. All researchers should identify the purpose of the research, and its aims or hypotheses, which will inform the choice of research paradigm and methodology chosen for the study.

Ethical considerations are fundamental to all research. Critiquing requires an appreciation of ethical principles, as well as consideration of how these are evidenced within the research process. A good discussion section of a paper should identify what the research has shown in relation to its original aims, as well as how these findings reflect what is already known about the subject and the policy context within which the research might be employed in nursing practice.

Activity: brief outline answer

Activity 3.2 Critical thinking (page 54)

The first way to quickly ascertain whether a paper is original research is to use the advanced filters that exist in some research engines to ensure that you identify only papers that are empirical research – these are often known as original papers. The second important method is to read the abstract, which will often identify a research aim or question, the methodology used, sampling method applied, data-collection methods used and the key findings, as well as the conclusions of the study. If the elements mentioned here are missing, chances are it is not a research paper.

Further reading

Cathala, X and Moorley, C (2018) How to appraise quantitative research. *Evidence-based Nursing*, 21 (4): 99–101. Available at: http://dx.doi.org/10.1136/eb-2018-102996

This paper provides a brief guide to critiquing quantitative research.

Ellis, P (2022) *Understanding Research for Nursing Students* (5th edn). London: Sage.

This book provides a structured introduction to research approaches and methods.

Gerrish, K and Lathlean, J (2015) *The Research Process in Nursing* (7th edn). Oxford: Wiley-Blackwell.

Chapter 3 on research ethics is an interesting read.

Moorley, C and Cathala, X (2019) How to appraise qualitative research. *Evidence-Based Nursing*, 22 (1): 10–13. Available at: http://dx.doi.org/10.1136/ebnurs-2018-103044

This paper provides a brief guide to critiquing qualitative research.

Moule, P (2021) *Making Sense of Research in Nursing, Health and Social Care* (7th edn). London: Sage.

Chapter 11 on critical appraisal and Appendix 1, a critical appraisal framework, are particularly helpful.

Parahoo, K (2014) *Nursing Research: Principles, Process and Issues* (3rd edn). London: Palgrave Macmillan.

Chapter 17 on critiquing research is very helpful.

Useful websites

https://casp-uk.net/

The Critical Appraisal Skills Programme has lots of documents to help critically appraise research including a number of methodologically specific checklists.

www.consort-statement.org

A structured and helpful website that demonstrates clearly strategies for creating research.

www.hra.nhs.uk

This is the home of the Human Research Authority for the UK.

https://jbi.global/critical-appraisal-tools

The Joanna Briggs Institute has a variety of critical appraisal tools available for use which relate to specific research methodologies.

Chapter 4 · Critiquing research: approach-specific elements

Peter Ellis

Chapter aims

After reading this chapter, you will be able to:

- demonstrate an understanding of the important issues for critiquing qualitative research;
- demonstrate an understanding of the important issues for critiquing quantitative research;
- identify the choices for the different research methods used in qualitative and quantitative research and be able to critique them;
- describe what good data analysis might look like when critiquing research.

Introduction

The purpose of this chapter is to explore in more depth the critical appraisal processes applied when critiquing qualitative or quantitative research. The distinction between the two research approaches (or paradigms) has already been made. This chapter will enable you to decipher what good research practice looks like within each of these paradigms and describe some of the reasons for the practical choices made about methodologies and methods within each approach, as well as developing a sense of what alternative research approaches might look like.

The chapter is split into two sections, the first dealing with qualitative research and the second with quantitative research. It complements the critiquing framework in the Appendix to this book, and together they identify the questions you might ask of research and some of the answers you might expect from a good paper. As in the previous chapter, there are a number of examples of research included within the text. You may find it useful to have some of these to hand when reading this chapter so that you can engage in critical appraisal of them as you read. Remember as you read this chapter that critiquing is not all about being negative; critique implies identifying the positive aspects of a paper, as well as identifying and justifying alternative approaches the researchers might have chosen. The art of research critiquing is therefore about identifying the strengths, weaknesses and alternative approaches that might be applied to a research study with a view to considering its value in informing your practice. As stated elsewhere in the book, developing as an evidence-based practitioner is about developing the skills, knowledge and attributes that enable you to question what you see around you in a meaningful way, using what you discover to guide your day-to-day nursing activity.

It is important that you understand the research process in order to be able to critique it. To this end, we strongly suggest that you acquire a number of research textbooks to support your learning and from which to reference your critique. As we shall see later, a good critique will identify something about the research, apply the correct research term to the issue, reference a definition of the term (using a research methods textbook) and then apply the learning about the term to the paper being critiqued. So, for example, you might identify that a question used in a piece of research is ambiguous; you will identify that this affects the validity of the question; you will define validity as the ability of a data-collection technique to measure what it is supposed to be measuring; you may come to the conclusion that the research question has perhaps not been satisfactorily answered and that the research lacks validity (at least in this element). Remember that when we use a technical word for the first time, it appears in **bold** type. This signifies that the word is used in the Glossary at the end of the book. If you don't understand a technical word, it is helpful to look it up in the Glossary where you will see a concise definition.

Critiquing qualitative research

Within this section we will explore the critiquing of qualitative research. Remember, qualitative research asks questions about people's experiences, attitudes, feelings, understandings and opinions. The qualitative paradigm is associated with the social sciences and 'people-focused' enquiry; it looks at the world from the point of view of the people who are experiencing or have experienced whatever it is the research is exploring. On the whole, approaches to qualitative research are inductive – that is, they start from a position of neutrality, ask a question and allow the answer to emerge as the research progresses; they allow what they observe to lead to the generation of a hypothesis, an idea or an understanding.

Qualitative research, therefore, is concerned with describing and understanding human experiences as they occur and are interpreted in real life. In critiquing, qualitative research attention focuses on the **credibility** of the evidence presented as an authentic account and accurate interpretation of the respondents' viewpoints in relation to the research questions being explored. This is in contrast to the attempts within quantitative research to find *the* answer to a given question.

The choice of methodology

We identified in Chapter 3 that the research paradigm upon which a research paper is based has to do with the school of thought that informs it. Methodologies are a more detailed plan of action used to undertake the research – the road map, if you like. Within qualitative research, the different methodologies provide a structure for undertaking the research and are selected because of how well they actually fit the question asked.

Research summary: choice of methodology

For their study of sexuality and childbearing in women living with HIV, Carlsson-Lalloo et al. (2018) identify the purpose of phenomenological research as explaining *a world with meanings, where people experience and share the world in relation to each other. There is no thinking that is separate from the body, but the body, subject and the world are intertwined. The so-called intersubjective world is accessed through the lived body, which is embedded and manifests itself through the lived experiences.* Phenomenology *contains methodological principles [such] as openness, flexibility and bridling …bridling [being] a methodological principle where the researchers need to embody a phenomenological attitude, which means adopting an openness and flexibility towards the explored phenomenon …* . Therefore, this design allows *what is not directly visible [to] become visible.*

(Continued)

> *It includes restraining one's pre-understanding and avoiding the act of defining what is undefinable* (p2). While this is a perfectly reasonable explanation of, and reason for using, phenomenology for this study, a number of other qualitative methodologies could have been used instead. Given that they want to 'describe the phenomenon [of] sexuality and childbearing as experienced by women living with HIV in Sweden' rather than, say, generate 'theoretical understanding of', the methodology fits the aim of the study as stated (Ellis, 2022a).

Many qualitative research papers do not identify a specific research methodology – they are called **generic** or **exploratory qualitative studies.** This is not, usually, a mistake on the part of the researchers; rather, it is a practical response to the fact that the question they are asking does not fit neatly into one of the established methodologies. In a critique, it is often sufficient to point this out and perhaps suggest a methodology that might have been chosen or, alternatively, a means of adjusting the question to make it potentially fit a particular approach with the best critiques suggesting both tweaks to the question and methodologies that fit these. So, for example, a qualitative study of student nurses' understandings of research (an exploratory or generic study) could be tweaked to become a **grounded theory** study that sought to generate a theory to understand student nurses' understandings of research.

Table 4.1 shows the main research methodologies used in qualitative research and gives some idea of the type of issues they are used to study.

Research methodologies are, therefore, the overall scheme by which research is undertaken, and the choice of methodology is driven by the exact research question being asked. For example, a question about what it is like to work in an oncology unit, caring for people with cancer, suggests the use of **ethnography**, while understanding the essence of how people cope with life with cancer will suggest that the study methodology should be **phenomenological**.

Methodology	What it studies
Ethnography	Studies cultures and groups and how they interact.
Grounded theory	Generates or develops a theory about a social interaction.
Phenomenology	Describes the essence or perceived reality of an experience/ intersubjective lived experiences.
Case study research	Explores case(s) of interest.
Generic qualitative	Studies people's attitudes, beliefs, opinions or experiences.

Table 4.1 Potential areas for study and their associated qualitative methodologies

When critiquing the choice of methodology for a piece of research, it is worth looking at the sometimes subtle differences between the methodologies and perhaps suggesting, rather than categorically stating, how a slightly modified question might have led the researchers to have used a different methodology. Where the methodology chosen appears to fit well with the question being asked, it is important to state why this is the case, as in the example critique earlier. One good method of checking how a topic could be researched is to look at other papers which have examined the same, or similar, topics to see what they have done (and how they have framed their questions); you might find some examples in the literature review/background section of the paper you are critiquing (and their references in the list at the end of the paper).

Sampling

When critiquing the choice of sampling method(s) and sample size in qualitative research, it is worth remembering what qualitative research seeks to do. Qualitative research seeks to inform the thinking about a topic and for its findings to be potentially **transferable** to other similar situations. This means that the findings are not said to be directly applicable – generalisable – to other similar situations, but they might inform decision-making – especially where the findings are supported by other, similar research.

In **biographic** and **case study research**, the sample may be as few as one individual rising up to dozens in ethnographic research. Most qualitative research methodologies – for example, phenomenological or grounded theory research – use sample sizes of between 6 and 15 participants, although this is open to justification by the authors and may also be determined by their findings as they progress through the study.

There are a number of characteristics of qualitative sampling that relate it to the purpose of the topic being studied. Since most qualitative research is about understanding individuals' perceptions and experiences, sampling involves identifying individuals who have had the experience that is being studied. Selecting people because they have had the experience of interest is called **purposive sampling** (Pope and Mays, 2020).

Because the individuals within the sample are similar on account of the shared experience, the sample may also be said to be **homogeneous**. In qualitative research, this is seen as a good feature of the research design, so long as the people selected represent the sorts of people the research question is about.

Homogeneous and purposive sampling means that the findings of qualitative research may be transferable to other similar people in similar situations and contexts – **transferability**. It is worth noting, however, that just because a sample is said to be homogeneous, this does not mean the interpretation of the experience will be the same for all concerned. Homogeneity in this sense relates to having experienced the same phenomenon; clearly, interpretation of the phenomenon, the individual's own reality, will vary from participant to participant.

Concept summary: purposive sampling

Purposive sampling refers to the fact that individuals are selected because they fit the purpose of the study – their purpose is to be able to talk about whatever experience is being studied. Individuals within such samples are also similar in that they share an experience or some other feature(s) in common; this is referred to as homogeneity, which literally means being the same – at least in respect of one important **variable**. However, this does not mean that they view the experience in the same way necessarily. When critiquing qualitative samples it is desirable that the characteristics of the individuals in a sample are identified to the reader and that you can understand who has been selected for the study and why. Understanding the characteristics and context of the research aids the reader in understanding how transferable the findings of the study might be to the place that they work and the people that they work with.

Many qualitative studies select participants from groups of individuals who are easily identified and handy to approach. These **convenience samples**, as they are called, are an acceptable way of recruiting participants to study (Creswell and Creswell, 2018). When such samples contain individuals who may be vulnerable, it is good practice to show within the sampling how this has been accounted for. Strategies may include approaching the individuals through a third party (such as another member of staff that they know or a relative or friend), seeking consent via a partner or close relative, or just excluding people who lack the ability to consent freely from the study.

Vulnerability may also lie in dependent relationships between the researcher and the subject – for example, a nurse and patient, or a lecturer and student. Care will need to be exercised in the consent process in such circumstances to avoid claims of coercion. Again, using a third party to request and gain consent from people in these circumstances is good practice and would be worthy of a positive comment in any critique.

Example critique: purposive and convenience sampling

In their study which sought to understand the experiences of family caregivers looking after people with end-stage kidney disease undergoing in-centre haemodialysis during the COVID-19 pandemic, Sousa et al. (2022) selected a purposive sample of people caring for a relative undergoing haemodialysis. The sample was also convenient in that all of the participants were drawn from people who were relatives of patients being dialysed within one of two dialysis units – in this respect they were easy to identify and were convenient to recruit via the head nurses of the units. Some ethical questions arise as to the burden of research placed on the participants and whether they felt obliged to participate in this research because their loved one was undergoing haemodialysis in the unit which identified them as a carer.

Activity 4.1   Reflection

Reflect on how you respond to approaches for help or information from different people – e.g., family and friends, your lecturers or the ward manager. What factors influence the responses that you give and in what situations do you feel more obliged to comply with the request? How might this reflect in the ways that people respond to requests to become involved in research in the hospital or other clinical setting?

An outline answer is provided at the end of the chapter.

Many qualitative studies use the point of **data saturation** as an idealised way of determining the size of the sample to be studied. Data from the interview or focus groups are analysed as the study progresses, and recruitment stops when no new ideas are emerging from the data – that is, when the data is saturated (Hennink and Kaiser, 2019). This is a reasonable approach to use in qualitative research and may be positively critiqued.

One other common approach to sampling, which is frequently used in grounded theory, is called **theoretical sampling** (Glaser and Strauss, 1967). Theoretical sampling occurs when the researcher has analysed early interviews within the study and has started to create some initial theories. This analysis leads the researcher to ask additional questions and prompts them to purposively recruit further participants to the study who are suitable to help answer emerging questions or to firm up the emerging theory. This is an extension of the idea of data saturation and makes good sense within qualitative methodologies that are inductive – that is, that allow the findings to emerge from the study as the data are collected, rather than starting with a preconceived idea as to what the findings might be, as may be the case with a quantitative study.

The best qualitative research papers will therefore identify the characteristics of their sample, the recruitment and sampling method used, as well as demonstrating how they have tried to go about this process in an ethical manner.

The choice of data-collection methods

Methods refer to the tools used to collect the data for a research project. When critiquing data-collection methods within qualitative research, it is important, as ever, to bear in mind the purpose of the research (which arises from the research question), the chosen methodology, and the capabilities and vulnerabilities of the people being researched. The nature of the research question will strongly determine the sense of the data-collection method being used.

Within qualitative research there are four main approaches to data collection: interviews, focus groups, observation and examination of artefacts (Ellis, 2022a). The choice of the data-collection method will relate strongly not only to the topic under investigation, but also to the characteristics of the participants.

For example, it might be reasonable to question the logic of a qualitative study that enquired into the nature of a potentially embarrassing topic (such as sexually transmitted diseases) using a focus group. It is clearly more appropriate (regardless of the methodology) to ask such questions in a one-to-one interview.

Example critique: data collection using focus groups

In their study examining abuse and mistreatment of women by healthcare workers in maternity settings in Kenya, Warren et al. (2017) used focus groups to collect some of their data. In consideration of some of the sensitivities of the subject under discussion, they used same-sex staff to run the groups. They also made it plain to participants that while the focus group was being taped, no personal identifiers (such as names) were being collected. Rather than suggest that there were problems in the maternity facilities with abuse, Warren et al. (2017) avoided biasing the discussions by framing the data collection as a general discussion about the experience of using maternity services. Some women who identified as having suffered abuse were then invited to have one-to-one interviews, as were a number who had not identified as experiencing abuse.

Where there are potential power relationships, or when individuals may be vulnerable in other ways, it may not be appropriate to use focus groups or observations to collect qualitative data, even if methodologically this is the preferred data-collection method. In these instances, the usefulness of the chosen methods has to take second place to the ethical principles of avoiding harm and respecting autonomy.

Activity 4.2   Critical thinking

In what sorts of situations might you feel less able to speak your mind than others? Why is this and why might this answer help you to understand how research participants view data-collection methods in qualitative research?

There are some possible answers at the end of the chapter.

Observational data collection may be a benefit in studies seeking to find out what people do or how they behave in certain situations. The use of observation may not be the correct method when the purpose of the study is to understand an issue from the perspective of the participant. Observation just does not fit the purpose – it is used to see what people do rather than study what they think. Observation followed by interviews or a focus group discussion, however, may be an appropriate choice of method when the research is seeking to find out what people do and then to understand why they do it in a particular situation.

In some research methodologies – for example, ethnograph – there is a clear need for the use of multiple methods of data collection. Ethnography seeks to understand the culture (beliefs, shared understandings and values), as well as the behaviours within a group; this requires a mix of observation, participation in the group and interviews (Parahoo, 2014). Some ethnography may also include the examination of artefacts, such as pictures and letters, in an effort to understand their meaning to the group. Failure to undertake at least two levels of data collection within ethnography would give cause for concern and raise questions about the completeness of the data collection – a very necessary and valid point for critique in this methodology.

Some questions around data collection in the qualitative methodologies are more subtle. For example, there remain questions about the use of semi-structured interviews in phenomenology where the consensus view used to be that the interviews should be unstructured (so that the respondent can shape the direction of the conversation). In many critical appraisals it would be reasonable to point this out without committing to one argument or the other.

Critiquing qualitative research methods, therefore, requires the reviewer to make some judgement about the justification the researcher has made for their choice of methods, or critiquing the absence of a justification. It also requires the reviewer to ask questions of themselves about what approach they would use when trying to obtain the same sorts of information from people in similar circumstances.

The analysis and results

The data that are produced in qualitative research are words. These words need sorting, grouping and interpreting in order to help make sense of the data collected for a study. There are several stages that can add credibility and **rigour** to this process and demonstrate the researcher's commitment to producing research findings that are transparent and high quality.

Concept summary: credibility and rigour

Credibility refers to how believable a piece of qualitative research is. The use of the term in relation to qualitative research suggests that the research undertaken actually answers what it set out to answer because of the quality of the way in which the research has been done.

Rigour in qualitative research suggests that the research process has been undertaken in a well thought through, fully explained and transparent manner. It also requires this is fully explained to those reading the paper.

There is no single right way in which to examine qualitative data. What is always important in qualitative data analysis is that the process is well explained and the decisions made in the process appear logical and transparent (credible and rigorous). This transparency requires the paper to explain exactly how the data were analysed and by whom, and what strategies they put in place to confirm the conclusions they came to.

It should be apparent that the study has been conducted in a neutral manner and the findings have been allowed to emerge – that is, the whole research process has been inductive and not based on confirming a pre-existing hypothesis. This neutrality of the data analysis process is said to bring **confirmability** to the study (Polit and Beck, 2020).

Commonly, papers will say that the author(s) read and reread the data (usually **verbatim** transcripts of interviews or focus groups) looking for common ideas and themes (termed **thematic analysis**) identifying the issues that were most important to the participants. This is a reasonable approach to data analysis, although many qualitative researchers are now using computer programs. What is important in critiquing the analysis of qualitative research is not so much the strategy used, but the supplementary strategies used to check the credibility and trustworthiness of this initial data analysis approach.

Key among the strategies used to confirm the findings of a study is the use of a second person to review the data collected – be they transcripts of interviews or focus groups, video or notes from observations of other artefacts – and come to their own conclusions about the findings. There may be some discussion about how a consensus view about the study results were then arrived at. A good study should explain this process in enough detail for the reader to understand what was done, by whom and when, so the reader is content about both the rigour and credibility of the analysis process.

The best studies using a single method (such as interviews or focus groups) will further check and report on the credibility of their findings in one of two ways. The first is to return the results to some, if not all, of the participants asking the question, 'Is this interpretation of the interview a good representation of what you said?' This strategy is sometimes called **member checking** or **respondent validation**, although more recent methodological advances include providing the opportunity for respondents to add to or alter what they said in interview up to several months after the interview in a process called **synthesised member checking**, which, it is claimed, aids the process of co-constructing knowledge in which the researcher engages in with participants (Birt et al., 2016).

The second approach is to present the findings to other researchers, or people with a special knowledge of the area of investigation, an expert panel, who are encouraged to ask probing questions about the methods used and the findings arrived at (Polit and Beck, 2020). Failure to do either of these might lead to some critical discussion in the critique.

In studies employing more than one data-collection method, the consistency of the findings between the different data-collection methods may be used to demonstrate the degree of credibility of the research. Where more than one data collector is used or different approaches employed, the study should demonstrate a consistency in the data collection; this is termed **dependability**. Dependability might be improved by ensuring that the data collectors are trained together so that they approach data collection in the same way.

A further strategy that helps the reader understand and perhaps come to some agreement with the findings of qualitative research is the use of verbatim (that is, word-for-word) quotes from the participants of the research alongside the themes and categories identified by the researcher. This allows the reader to understand how they have arrived at the findings they have and to develop an awareness of why the researchers have come to the conclusions they have. Clearly, the interpretation of what a research participant has said relies to some extent on the context of the conversation in which they said it; nevertheless, verbatim quotes give the critical reviewer a view into the world of the research participant that is missing in studies that do not use them.

Example critique: establishing credibility

In their study of the lived experiences of women with cervical cancer in Uganda, Natuhwera et al. (2021) used semi-structured interviews for data collection. Three researchers independently analysed the data and derived their own themes, which were then compared and a consensus reached. Verbatim quotes are presented in the article to help validate the themes. While both of these strategies are useful in helping demonstrate rigour and credibility, there is no real information about the process undertaken when the researchers met to discuss the emerging themes, nor does it appear that participants were asked to verify the themes. While neither of these issues mean that the study is poor, they are both worth a mention in any critique.

While the findings of qualitative research are not said to be generalisable (necessarily applicable) to other people similar to the participants, the existence in the discussion of other similar research showing similar findings demonstrates that the study has some transferability to other groups of individuals.

Critiquing quantitative research

Quantitative research is research that uses numbers and statistics; it is concerned with cause and effect, exposures and outcomes. Key among the concerns for quantitative research are that it should be **valid**, **reliable** and **generalisable**.

Concept summary: validity, reliability and generalisability

Validity is the ability of a data-collecting tool (a method) to measure what it is supposed to be measuring. For example, we know that a sphygmomanometer (when used properly) will measure blood pressure; however, it is much more difficult to know how well a questionnaire designed to measure anxiety levels actually does so because it may be hard to define what anxiety is. In many studies of anxiety and stress the data collected from questionnaires are supplemented by taking biological samples and measuring the level of cortisol (a hormone associated with stress) in them, as a way of validating the findings.

Reliability refers to the reproducibility of the results of the study. Reliability may refer to whether the data-collection tool (such as a questionnaire) produces broadly similar results when used again in the same population, when applied to the same sample at a different time or when the tool is used by another researcher.

Generalisability refers to the extent to which the findings from a piece of research can be extended out to the general population of people in a similar position – that is, whether the sample used in the research is representative enough of the population to which the findings of the research are to be applied.

Many quantitative studies focus on answering a question that is posed as a hypothesis, which we described earlier as being an idea that can be tested using the scientific method. By their nature, quantitative studies are therefore **deductive**, setting out to answer the question of the research using a methodology and methods best suited to establishing the truth, or otherwise, of the initial hypothesis.

The choice of methodology

As with all research, the methodology (which is the broad plan of action for the study) has to fit the questions being asked. The wrong choice of methodology means that a study cannot answer the questions it set out to answer. When critiquing the choice of methodology, it is important to understand what each of the different methodologies can be used to research. For example, cause and effect can only be examined with any confidence in experimental studies (which include randomised controlled trials) and cohort studies, as these are both **prospective** and **longitudinal** – that is, they collect data as things happen over a period of time. Quantitative methods that are not both prospective and longitudinal cannot make this claim, as they do not collect data in a forward-going real-time manner and do not establish whether the outcome of interest was present at the start of the study.

Table 4.2 shows the sorts of questions that the various quantitative methodologies can be used to answer.

Questions	Methodology
If x is done, what will happen? If x is done, how often will y happen?	Experiment/quasi-experiment/randomised controlled trial.
If a person is exposed to x, will they develop outcome (disease) y? Does exposure to x cause outcome y?	Cohort studies.
What exposure x might have caused this individual to have outcome y?	Case-control studies.
In this group of people, how many have been exposed to x or have outcome y? What is the prevalence of x or y in this group?	Cross-sectional studies.
The data show that when x increases in the population, so too does y. Might they be associated? When exposure x increases and outcome y increases, is there potential that the two are associated in some way?	Ecological studies.

Table 4.2 Questions that different quantitative methodologies can be used to answer

Source: Ellis, 2022a.

While Table 4.2 is not an exhaustive list of the quantitative methodologies, it provides some clarity as to what the different methods can do. In terms of critiquing the choice of quantitative research methodologies, perhaps the most important question is whether the chosen approach is suitable for examining cause-and-effect relationships.

This is perhaps best understood by remembering that all quantitative methodologies are concerned with the quality of the measurement of variables, where variables are any factors within a study that may differ (vary) between study participants. The quality of the measurements, and therefore the validity and reliability of the study, relies heavily on the elimination of bias within the research process.

Concept summary: bias

Bias is defined as a deviation from the truth. Bias occurs when a deviation from the truth is the result of defects in the way in which a study is carried out. For example, **recall bias** occurs where a study relies on the memory of participants – for example, remembering what they ate last week, recalling their alcohol intake over a period of time or whether or not they have ever had chickenpox.

Because in the examples given these variables are not being measured in real time (prospectively) or over a period of time (longitudinally) or, indeed, in a standardised way (which will affect both validity and reliability), there is a degree of uncertainty about how good the quality of the data collected actually is. Significantly, bias can mean that a study is fatally flawed and its findings are of no value; consequently, quantitative researchers expend a lot of time and energy trying to design bias out of their studies.

Taking these issues into account identifies why studies that seek to prove cause and effect need to be prospective and longitudinal, while those that seek only to measure the amount of a certain variable or demonstrate an association or correlation (which conceptually are not as strong as demonstrating cause-and-effect relationships) do not.

Example critique: choice of methodology

Lopez Salguero and Andrés Collado (2018) determined to identify the characteristics of gout, which may be associated with an increased risk of cardiovascular disease. They chose a case control study because they were not looking for a cause-and-effect relationship, but rather only an association. Using a case control approach allowed them to examine various elements of gout and identify whether these 'cases' also had cardiovascular disease. The study is strengthened by the fact that they excluded people from the study who had proven cardiovascular disease before they had gout. They further added credence to their findings that time since the first attack of gout and the presence of gout in a number of joints, both associated with a high degree of inflammation, were associated with a higher burden of cardiovascular disease – persistent inflammation being an emerging area of interest among risk factors for cardiovascular disease in many other studies. When critiquing the choice of methodology, therefore, it is important to identify the expressed purpose (aims and objectives) of the study and the level of proof associated with it, which will determine the choice of research methodology. Identifying the purpose of the study will indicate whether the methodology needs to be prospective and longitudinal or not. A good critique will pick up on this and might express that the choice of study methodology is a good one, a poor one or that alternative methodologies might also have been chosen.

Sampling

When thinking about the quality of the sampling methods applied in quantitative research, it is important to remember that the key purpose of this form of enquiry is to produce data that are generalisable – that is to say, quantitative studies seek to produce results that can be applied beyond the sample in which the study took place. To be generalisable, therefore, quantitative studies need to have samples that are **representative** of people who are broadly similar to all the people the study is about.

Concept summary: representativeness

Representativeness is about the degree to which the study sample is comparable to the population from which it was taken – for example, in relation to gender, age, ethnicity and severity of disease. The more typical the sample is with regard to the population the study is about, the more likely the findings of the study hold true in that population (generalisability). In this sense, population refers to people with a similar characteristic – for example, being a student nurse, and not the wider population as a whole.

In terms of critiquing, this means that the sample used for the study should represent the sorts of people who are identified in the study question. For example, a study of the understanding of dietary management among people newly diagnosed with diabetes should identify what it means by diabetes (Type 1 or Type 2), as well as what it means by newly diagnosed (say, in the last six months). The selection of potential participants for the study would then be focused on all people who fit these criteria; this would be termed the **study population**.

In some research, all the people in this population might be studied, especially when the population is drawn from a small geographic area or from people with a rare disease – assuming they all gave their consent to participate. Studies that employ this type of sample might include **cross-sectional studies**.

In more sophisticated studies, such as experimental studies, the selection of people from a large potential study population allows everyone the same chance of being included in the study. This is called **probability sampling** and produces a **study sample**. If the sample size is large enough (as calculated using statistical formulae), it can produce a sample that is representative of the larger population, and hence generalisable results.

Where a paper does not identify the processes that occurred in relation to forming the study sample, there are questions that need to be asked about the quality of the sampling, the potential for the introduction of bias and therefore about how generalisable the findings of such research can be.

Activity 4.3   Critical thinking

If someone were to undertake a study looking at stress in nurses, consider how many of your colleagues, and from which branches of nursing, they might need to sample in order to get a reasonable understanding of this issue. Consider what impression they might form of stress in nursing if they were to interview just one or two of your colleagues perhaps directly after a night shift, after a busy day or following a death on the ward.

An outline answer is provided at the end of the chapter.

In **randomised controlled trials** (RCTs), the process goes a step further. Because RCTs seek to examine the difference in outcomes between two or more similar groups to investigate the effectiveness of an intervention, there is a need for the two groups to be broadly similar at the start of the study – or any findings made could be claimed to be the result of the differences between the groups rather than the results of the intervention being studied. So, in an RCT you would expect to see that the study sample is further divided into cases (participants to whom the intervention/study drug is given) and controls (participants who get a dummy intervention or drug) (Ellis, 2022a). This process must happen randomly (to avoid introducing **selection bias** to the study) and all good RCTs will identify how this is achieved.

Example critique: randomised sample

In their study of the usefulness of an eight-week course in mindfulness for reducing stress, Galante et al. (2018) randomised student participants using a remote survey software which generated random numbers. The method ensured that there were equal numbers of participants in each arm. Notably, the student participants self-assessed themselves as having no mental health issue at the start of the study period. Which arm of the study the students were in and whether they were undertaking the course or not was concealed from the researchers and outcomes assessors. In terms of critique, self-assessment of one's mental health status may not be all that accurate and this sort of study may attract people who are struggling to cope with and conceal existing mental health issues. The fact that outcome data was also collected remotely did allow for the randomisation status of the student to remain hidden from the research team even in the absence of a **sham intervention**.

In some cases where the splitting of the groups cannot happen randomly, there remain questions about the quality of the research process, especially around the introduction of bias. While it would be correct to critique this element of the research, allowances have to be made where the decision not to create the groups randomly was a practical consideration – for example, when it is hard to hide from the participants and the researchers which group the individual participant has been allocated to – for example, when using a particular type of wound dressing.

In case-control studies, the selection of cases is based on them having the outcome (usually a disease) of interest, with controls being similar in as many other respects as possible – for example, age, gender, ethnicity, income group and educational attainment. In matched cohort studies, the controls are chosen because they are similar to the cases being studied in as many respects as possible other than being exposed to the potential cause of the disease under study. In both types of study, it is the role of the researcher to create a convincing argument as to why they chose the control groups they did, and the best papers will identify the limitations of the study that arise from the compromises made in this process somewhere in the discussion. Regardless of whether the authors identify the limitation or not, the best critiques will identify and discuss these issues.

Many quantitative papers identify a starting sample but appear to report data from a smaller sample in the results. This is usually the result of losses to the study from people withdrawing for any number of reasons. It is reasonable to criticise a study in which this occurs when the reasons for, and the characteristics of, the withdrawals are not discussed. There are good reasons for this.

Some withdrawals may be related to some aspect of the thing being studied – for example, a side-effect of a drug. Significant numbers of withdrawals from a study because of a side-effect may not have statistical, but may have important clinical implications. Withdrawal of certain groups of people from the study, perhaps older patients or those of a particular gender, may mean that the findings of the study are skewed and that they can no longer claim to be generalisable. Clearly, in a study of two arms such as an RCT, significant withdrawals from the treatment arm may mean that the new drug or intervention is unacceptable to many people and may not be as clinically successful as the researchers suggest. This is worthy of an unambiguous negative critique.

The choice of data-collection methods

We have already made the assertion that all quantitative methodologies are concerned with the quality of the measurement of variables. Nowhere within the quantitative research process is this more obvious than in the choice of data-collection methods. Essentially, there are two elements to data-collection methods that are open to potential critique. The first is the actual choice of the tool itself and its potential to be able to measure whatever it is that it is trying to measure – its validity. Second is the issue of how the tool is actually put to work, how reliable the way in which it was used is.

The most frequently used data-collection tools in nursing research are questionnaires and other forms of surveys. In many cases the variables a study seeks to measure are already the subjects of well-tried and tested questionnaires, or other tools, the validity of which is well established. The best research papers will identify why they chose the questionnaire(s) and how well these might apply to the people they are studying. Poorer quality papers will identify what tools they used, but give little or no explanation as to why. A top tip for critiquing is to look up the tool online and see what other researchers might say about its strengths and weaknesses; the very best critiques might go so far as to identify alternative data-collection tools.

Activity 4.4   Research and finding out

A large number of questionnaires exist to measure diverse health and socially related variables in research. These data collection tools can be used to measure variables such as quality of life, mental well-being and levels of anxiety either generally or in relation to specific diseases. Go online and try to identify some of these and read about what it is they are designed to be able to measure. Spend some time trying to find some critiques of the strengths and weaknesses of the particular tool and alternative tools one might use to investigate a variable you are interested in – for example, quantifying pain. You may find this approach useful when critiquing a paper.

Some websites are identified at the end of this chapter where you could look at some validated questionnaires and data-collection tools.

Other data for quantitative studies may be collected from existing sources such as databases, and medical and nursing records. The quality of this data will vary greatly and the best studies will make allowances for this and may make some efforts to check the quality of both the data and the accuracy and consistency (reliability) of the collection of it for research purposes (especially where more than one person is used for data collection).

Physiological and biological data are frequently collected in quantitative studies. The quality of these forms of data is thought by many nurses to be beyond question; this is not, however, always the case. For example, blood pressure measurements, even when undertaken using the same apparatus, vary between individuals who are taking the measurement (especially where it is taken manually). The best quality research will try to minimise this difference by training all those involved to use the same method to take blood pressures and thereby increase reliability.

With regard to biological and physiological data, the best papers will record how specimens and measurements were taken, by whom, under what conditions, where, how often and how data-collection staff were trained. In some of the best research reports, there will be data on the degree of agreement between different data-collection staff, typically measured in statistical terms such as the **kappa statistic**. When critiquing, if this level of detail is missing it is worthy of comment.

The analysis and results

The analysis of quantitative research invariably requires the use of statistics. These statistics are of two separate kinds. The first are **descriptive statistics**, the purpose of which is to describe the study sample and perhaps some of the outcomes. The best research papers will contain descriptive statistics that explain the frequency, spread and measures of central tendency (for example, the **means** and **medians**) of the data. Such data should give you a good idea of some of the characteristics of the study participants, such as their ages and gender. In comparison studies, such as RCTs and matched cohorts, the reader should also be able to see that the two groups are broadly similar in all described variables at the start of the study. If they appear not to be, this would give cause for critique because difference at the start might give rise to differences at the end of the study which are unrelated to either the issue being studied or the intervention.

The second form of statistics used are what are referred to as **inferential statistics**. These statistics describe the levels of confidence that the researchers place in their findings and are derived from applying various statistical tests.

A large number of statistical tests can be applied to numerical data, and the best papers leave the reader in no doubt about what tests have been applied using which statistical packages. Clearly, it is beyond the scope of this text to delve into these now; however, there are many good guides that explain which statistical tests apply to which forms of data and in what circumstances.

Activity 4.5   Research and finding out

A large number of statistical tests can be applied to numerical data. Go online and try to identify some of these and read about what it is they are designed to do. You may find this strategy useful when critiquing a paper. You are advised to look up and understand in particular the nature and purpose of the t-test and the chi-squared test.

There are some websites identified at the end of this chapter where you could look at examples of statistics used with different forms of data.

The analysis and presentation of results within quantitative research can be quite confusing because of the numbers involved. The best papers will, however, present their findings in a variety of ways, including graphs, tables and charts, many of which are fairly simple to understand and interpret. It is not a matter for critique that the reader is not familiar with the approach to analysis employed. A good critique will involve the novice reader in learning some things about the basic elements of what they are reading and applying it.

Using critiquing tools

As well as the tool presented in this book, there are a number of other good and well-used tools that help the novice and more experienced researcher to critique research papers. Perhaps the best known of these are the Critical Appraisal Skills Programme (CASP) checklists identified in Chapter 1.

Activity 4.6   Research and finding out

Go online to the CASP website (listed at the end of the chapter) and identify the critiquing tools listed there which can be applied to various research approaches. It is worth taking one of these tools and using it to critique a research paper you are interested in – perhaps one of those identified in this chapter. Consider how the structure of the questions enables you to critique the paper in a considered and logical fashion. Consider bookmarking sites such as CASP so that you can return to them later and use them for your studies.

Getting used to using tools such as CASP checklists when looking at research will doubtless improve your ability both to critique and understand research better. As with all such tools, including the one contained in this book, you are advised to apply them alongside the use of a research textbook that will enable you to look up and understand terminology with which you are not familiar, as well as to read about how the best research is undertaken; a couple of good textbooks are listed at the end of the chapter.

Chapter summary

The approach to critiquing is driven by what the research ultimately aims to do. The choice of research methodology, and whether or not it is qualitative or quantitative, should have been informed by the exact questions, the nature of those questions and the type of person about whom the research seeks to find answers.

There are various approaches to identifying and recruiting samples for both qualitative and quantitative research, and these are decided by considering both theoretical and practical issues. Similarly, there are a number of different methods that can be used to collect data, and it is the role of the researcher to defend the choices they made.

As with all stages of the research process, the choice of data-collection method arises out of both theoretical and practical considerations. Researchers need to make it plain why they make the choices they do. While recognising this, a good critique may include some suggestions about why the method might or might not be the best choice, as well as suggestions for other methods of data collection.

The analysis of data is a process that needs justification in the qualitative paradigm, and explanation and transparency in both qualitative and quantitative research.

Activities: Brief outline answers

Activity 4.1 Reflection (page 71)

The ways in which we are approached and by whom certainly have an effect on the ways in which we respond to requests for help. We feel obligations to people who employ us, people we work with and our family. These obligations arise from a sense of duty, belonging and, in the case of family, love, and may conflict with our own true wishes. Approaches in person are harder to ignore, while those in writing or via e-mail may prove easier to ignore. While writing this answer, I was phoned by someone collecting for a charity I did not want to support; it was easy to say no on the phone, whereas face-to-face in the street I might spend more time over saying no.

Asking people who are patients to become involved in research may create dilemmas for them where they, too, feel a sense of obligation arising out of duty to respond to the care they have received, the desire to belong and please their carers, and perhaps affection and gratitude. As suggested in the text, this may mean that researchers have to explore ways for patient participants to exercise freedom of choice in relation to research, which may mean making it easy to say no or simply ignore a written request.

Activity 4.2 Critical thinking (p 72)

There are often potential issues within qualitative research that need to be accounted for in the choice of data-collection methods. These include power relationships between the researcher and the participant – and, indeed, between participants themselves. For instance, you may not feel able to talk openly about how you feel about your job in front of your boss, and you may not want to talk about your home life in front of your colleagues.

Similarly, participants in research are not likely to want to discuss certain issues in a focus group format, and if they do, they may choose not to be completely truthful, so the choice of method will impact on the credibility of the research findings.

Activity 4.3 Critical thinking (page 79)

If researchers were to interview only a couple of nurses as they came off a night shift, it is likely they would form the impression that nurses were all terribly stressed, or perhaps not. The impression they would form would be influenced almost entirely by what sort of night the two nurses had experienced; in this respect, it is influenced by the timing of the study and the fact only two nurses are involved. It might also be fair to say that the study only represented one type of nurse – e.g. adult nurses, and this, together with it being a small sample, means that it is not generalisable to all nurses.

Further reading

Bland, M (2015) *An Introduction to Medical Statistics* (4th edn). Oxford: Oxford University Press.

A really well-known and comprehensive beginners' guide to statistics.

Coughlan, M, Cronin, P and Ryan, F (2007) Step-by-step guide to critiquing research. Part 1: quantitative research. *British Journal of Nursing*, 16 (11): 658–63.

This is a reasonable overview of critiquing quantitative research.

Ellis, P (2022) *Understanding Research for Nursing Students* (5th edn). London: Sage.

A student's guide to research.

Parahoo, K (2014) *Nursing Research: Principles, Process and Issues* (3rd edn). London: Palgrave Macmillan.

Chapter 17 on critiquing research is very helpful.

Polit, DF and Tatano Beck, CT (2020) *Essentials of Nursing Research: Appraising Evidence for Nursing Research* (10th edn). London: Lippincott, Williams & Wilkins.

A very detailed book about nursing research methods.

Ryan, F, Coughlan, M and Cronin, P (2007) Step-by-step guide to critiquing research. Part 2: qualitative research. *British Journal of Nursing*, 16 (12): 738–44.

This is a reasonable overview of critiquing qualitative research.

Silverman, D (2022) *Doing Qualitative Research* (6th edn). London: Sage.

Among the best guides to undertaking qualitative research.

Useful websites

https://casp-uk.net/

The home of the Critical Appraisal Skills Programme, including a number of very usable checklists.

www.graphpad.com

Click on 'Resources' and explore the various headings in the statistics guide.

https://jbi.global/critical-appraisal-tools

The Joanna Briggs Institute has a variety of critical appraisal tools available for use which relate to specific research methodologies.

http://statpages.org

A very useful statistics resource.

Websites containing validated data-collection questionnaires:

www.rand.org/health/surveys_tools/mos/36-item-short-form.html

Short form 36 is widely used to measure self-reported quality of life and functionality.

http://survmeth.blogspot.com/2015/01/sources-for-survey-questions-and.html

An interesting site for questionnaire resources.

Chapter 5 Making sense of subjective experience

Mooi Standing

NMC Future Nurse: Standards of Proficiency for Registered Nurses

This chapter will address the following proficiencies:

Platform 1: Being an accountable professional

At the point of registration, the registered nurse will be able to:

1.10 demonstrate resilience and emotional intelligence and be capable of explaining the rationale that influences their judgments and decisions in routine, complex and challenging situations.
1.17 take responsibility for continuous self-reflection, seeking and responding to support and feedback to develop their professional knowledge and skills.

Platform 3: Assessing needs and planning care

At the point of registration, the registered nurse will be able to:

3.4 understand and apply a person-centred approach to nursing care, demonstrating shared assessment, planning, decision making and goal setting when working with people, their families, communities and populations of all ages.

Platform 4: Providing and evaluating care

At the point of registration, the registered nurse will be able to:

4.3 demonstrate the knowledge, communication and relationship management skills required to provide people, families and carers with accurate information that meets their needs before, during and after a range of interventions.

> ## Chapter aims
>
> By the end of this chapter, you should be able to:
>
> - explain subjective experience and emotional intelligence, giving examples;
> - relate inter-subjective understanding to evidence-based, person-centred care;
> - understand the need for researcher reflexivity in eliciting subjective experience;
> - apply reflexive awareness in identifying areas for personal/professional growth.

Introduction

This chapter attempts to explain how the elusive nature of subjective experience can and should be incorporated within evidence-based practice in nursing. In doing so, it identifies the important contribution subjective experience makes to the model on which this book is based: *The influences on and dispositions of an evidence-based nurse.* For example, the influences 'Experience' and 'Patient preferences', together with the dispositions 'Engaged with self' and 'Other regarding', are all manifestations of personal, subjective and interpersonal, intersubjective experience within patient-centred, evidence-based nursing and healthcare.

We start by defining subjective experience and discuss how it informs people's biographies and psychosocial development with reference to Erikson's theory. We consider how emotional intelligence and intersubjective understanding contribute to person-centred, evidence-based care. We then explore researcher reflexivity (with reference to Reinharz's 'three categories of selves') in accurately reporting respondents' subjective experience, and we also apply reflexive awareness to review our professional development needs as nurses.

What is subjective experience?

Being subjective is defined as: *based on personal opinion, thoughts, feelings, etc.; not impartial*, which is the opposite of being objective, defined as: *not depending on, or influenced by, personal opinions or prejudices; relating to external facts, etc. as opposed to internal thoughts or feelings* (Chambers, 2014). For example, our hopes and fears, likes and dislikes, emotions and values, ambitions and dreams, sense of self and perceptions of others are all subjective because they reflect our personal, individual points of view, whereas the neurotransmitters in our brains that enable us to think and feel, and the technological innovations we use to communicate or travel are objective because they apply impersonal and scientifically verifiable knowledge. **Subjective experience** is therefore the product of our unique individual biographies, personalities, conscious and unconscious minds, and sensory awareness as we interact with other people and the physical environment. The following scenario illustrates the highly personalised nature of subjective experience.

Scenario: 'It's raining on me!'

Victoria, age 3, is in the back garden playing on her own with a toy wheelbarrow while her mum is inside preparing lunch. She is engrossed in her gardening game and does not notice the sunshine giving way to dark clouds appearing overhead. Suddenly it starts to rain heavily, Victoria gets wet, stops playing, starts crying and quickly runs inside shouting, 'Mummy, mummy, mummy – it's raining on me!'

Three-year-old Victoria exemplifies the meaning of subjective experience when she says 'it's raining on me!' rather than simply saying 'it's raining'. In doing so, Victoria emphasises that the sudden downpour has a personal impact upon her, interrupting her private world of play, which she is unhappy and a bit indignant about, resulting in a behaviour change – abandoning her game, and seeking comfort and shelter. Of course, it wasn't just raining on Victoria, but it clearly felt that way to her at the time. As she grows up, her subjective experience will become less egocentric, incorporating greater awareness of others, understanding of the wider world and her place in it. However, the personal impact upon her of interacting with other people and the environment will remain a key factor in defining the nature of her subjective experiences throughout life.

Erik Erikson (1902–94), a psychoanalyst, devised a psychosocial theory of human development, explaining how we encounter a different psychosocial crisis at eight key stages, ranging from 'trust versus mistrust' in early infancy to 'integrity versus despair' in old age (Gross, 2020). How we each perceive and resolve these tensions and mature as individuals is affected by the quality of the relationships we form with significant others during our lives. The above scenario relates to Stage 3 'initiative versus guilt' where young children learn through play activities when they might re-enact things that they have observed family members doing – for example, Victoria's gardening game. Stage 5 'identity versus role confusion' in adolescence is a particularly testing time as we establish a sense of who we are and how to be ourselves beyond the relatively protected confines of home, school or neighbourhood. Stage 6 'intimacy versus isolation' in early adulthood focuses on our capacity to form and maintain meaningful personal, work-related, and social relationships with others. Our sense of purpose, self-esteem, confidence to take on new challenges, knowing who we can trust, maintenance of appropriate interpersonal boundaries, self-awareness, self-care ability and capacity to care for others are influenced by how we negotiate the eight stages of psychosocial development, according to Erikson's theory. Hence, at whatever point we are in the human life cycle, we perceive ourselves, others and the environmental context subjectively, according to our unique psychological characteristics, personal biographies and life experience. It is as though everything each of us experiences in life is filtered through our own bespoke imaginary spectacles that tend to focus on what we find personally significant and meaningful to us.

Activity 5.1   Reflection

This activity is to help you to relate the concept of subjective experience to yourself. Take some time to think about your own life up to this point. Use the framework to describe significant people, memorable incidents you experienced from childhood to adulthood, and the impact they had on you both then and now.

	Childhood	Adolescence	Adulthood
Significant people in my life at this time			
Memorable incident that had an effect on me			
Impact on me at the time regarding my feelings, thoughts and behaviour			
Any lasting impact on how I see myself now or how I relate to others			

Notice similarities or differences between the people involved, the nature of incidents and your reactions to them during different phases of your life to date. Recalling life experiences in this way offers a snapshot of your personal biography and associated frames of reference that inform your subjective view of the world.

As this activity is based on your own observations, there is no outline answer at the end of the chapter.

Subjective experience: part of evidence-based practice?

There are opposing views about the value and usefulness of exploring and interpreting subjective experience within evidence-based practice. The hierarchies of evidence described in Chapter 1 ascribe higher status to objective, quantifiable, statistical data from experimental research applying rigorous scientific methods. This approach is often used to record physiological changes, for example, when testing the effectiveness of new pharmacological treatments in controlled 'double-blind' clinical trials. Subjectivity is eliminated from this type of research design as far as possible through: 1) random selection of subjects/allocation to experimental or control groups; 2) reliable measurement tools; 3) statistical tests of significance and probability of data validity; and 4) independent verification of results to minimise bias (selection/respondent/measurement/confirmation) in research. By definition, subjective experience is personal, so it is not impartial and it is very difficult to observe directly or quantify because it focuses on psychological and social processes rather than physical reality. However, describing and making sense of people's opinions, feelings, interactions and subjective experience of health and illness, treatment and care is highly valued in qualitative research studies.

The model of evidence-based nursing used in this book (Figure 1.1) embraces a range of relevant research, whether it is quantitative or qualitative, and sources knowledge from patient preference, experience and professional opinion to health policy, ethical and legal requirements informing clinical decisions. It therefore values the contribution of both subjective experience and objective measures of observable, empirical data. The model's *Dispositions of an evidence-based nurse* reflect this balanced approach by including 'Other regarding', 'Engaged with self' (subjective) alongside 'Reflexive', 'Critical thinker' (objective) qualities. The model also emphasises that the whole point of evidence-based nursing is to help ensure the highest standards of patient-centred care. In other words, care that effectively addresses people's needs, preferences and the right to be treated safely, skilfully, effectively, humanely and without prejudice. The next case study highlights how challenging delivering person-centred, evidence-based nursing care can be.

Case study: Non-judgemental, evidence-based care of a suspected mass killer

On 27 October 2018, a 46-year-old truck driver with no previous criminal record walked into a synagogue in Pittsburgh, Pennsylvania, USA shouting 'All Jews must die', killing 11 people aged 54–97 (including two brothers with learning disabilities) with a rifle and three handguns that he legally owned. He wounded six others, including four police officers, and he also suffered multiple gunshot wounds. When he surrendered, he was taken to a local hospital for life-saving medical treatment under armed guard. The person in charge of the hospital, himself a Jew who attends the synagogue, later informed local news channels that a doctor and nurse who first attended to the truck driver's wounds were also Jews. The Jewish nurse was on duty in the Emergency Room (ER); he had heard about the shooting before the suspect arrived and was wondering whether his father (a Rabbi) and mother were safe. The incident reminded him of the anti-Semitic abuse he had suffered at school

(Continued)

(images of a family marched into a gas chamber drawn on his desk, swastikas drawn on his locker and messages left for him saying, 'Die Jew, love Hitler'). Despite this, he hurried to attend to the patient/prisoner when he was wheeled into ER shouting 'Death to all Jews'. The nurse's first priority was to assess the multiple gunshot wounds and apply compression devices to prevent further haemorrhaging; he then monitored vital signs: breathing, oxygen saturation, heart rate, blood pressure, level of consciousness; managed intravenous lines, fluids and blood transfusion; took care to prevent further injury or infection; managed pain control, and ensured nil by mouth in preparation for surgical repair of the patient's gunshot wounds. The nurse said he carried out his duties with kindness and compassion as he felt the best way to honour the victims was for a Jew to prove the alleged mass killer was wrong about them. He did not reveal that he was a Jew at the time and suspected the patient/prisoner had no idea that he was, because he thanked him for saving his life.

Activity 5.2   Critical thinking

Having read through the case study, give some thought to answering the following questions with reference to Figure 1.1: *The influences on and dispositions of an evidence-based nurse.*

1. What impact did caring for a suspected mass killer and hater of Jews have on the Jewish nurse?
2. What impact did being cared for by the nurse appear to have on the suspected mass killer?
3. How did the nurse apply the *Dispositions of an evidence-based nurse* to *practice?*
4. Which *Influences on practice* provided evidence to support the nurse's actions?
5. How effectively were the principles of person-centred care applied to practice?
6. How might the nurse's biography/psychosocial development have influenced his career choice?

Some possible answers can be found at the end of the chapter.

The case study illustrates the continuous interplay between subjective experience and the more objective indicators of physical reality. Clearly, the main focus was urgent, life-saving physical intervention, but it also involved forming a non-judgemental, caring relationship with someone the nurse had every reason to fear. In doing so, the nurse demonstrated 'resilience and emotional intelligence' (NMC proficiency 1.10 – start of chapter) to carry out his professional duty of care in very difficult circumstances. It also suggests that developing understanding of subjective experience and human relationships is no less important than any scientific discoveries and technological advancements in relation to person-centred, evidence-based nursing.

Person-centred, inter-subjective emotional intelligence

Registered nurses need to *understand and apply a person-centred approach to nursing care* (NMC proficiency 3.4 – start of chapter) which is reinforced in *The Code: Professional standards of practice and behaviour for nurses and midwives* (NMC, 2018b, p6) that requires us to:

> *Prioritise people – You put the interests of people using or needing nursing or midwifery services first. You make their care and safety your main concern and make sure their dignity is preserved and their needs are recognised, assessed and responded to. You make sure that those receiving care are treated with respect, that their rights are upheld and that any discriminatory attitudes and behaviours towards those receiving care are challenged.*

We cannot put this into practice if we just assume that we know what patients need from their medical diagnosis. For example, they are likely to feel anxious and might be unclear about the nature of their health problems, proposed treatments, and the short- or possible long-term effects on their lives and relationships with others. In a survey asking patients to describe in three words 1) their experience of being a patient, and 2) the impact their illness had on their lives, they answered: 1) *frustrating, frightened* and *vulnerable;* and 2) *tiredness, discomfort* and *worry* (Patients Association, 2020). The Patients Association argues that it is important to define a patient as someone living with a health or care need rather than simply someone who is a recipient of healthcare services. The former is more person-centred, while the latter is more service-centred in its conceptualisation of patients. If we manage to elicit and understand the everyday lived experience of patients in our care, we are better informed about them as individuals with particular health needs, together with their perceptions of the care that they are receiving. In other words, patients have a better subjective understanding of what an illness or disease process feels like than the healthcare practitioners who look after them – we can only measure the signs of disease, but need patients to tell us what the symptoms are. Health knowledge is not therefore exclusive to professionals who have an understanding of the objective nature of illness and injury, and associated clinical expertise. Patients may also be considered 'experts by experience' regarding the impact of health problems on their lives now and in the future (Skilton et al., 2020). Hence, it is important that nurses try to tap into patients' subjective understanding in order to identify how they view their health problems, care plans and nursing interventions.

Person-centred care therefore depends on nurses applying good listening and communication skills so that patients can express any concerns they may have, seek clarification as necessary, express their preferences in contributing to care plans, and feel treated as valued partners in collaborative clinical decision-making to address their health issues (Standing, 2020). In this way, the subjective worlds of patient and nurse can establish a meaningful connection or 'meeting of minds' through intersubjective understanding, enabling nurses to empathise with patients, which informs effective, person-centred, evidence-based nursing.

Intersubjective understanding involves **emotional intelligence (EI)** as well as Intellectual Quotient (IQ) because subjective experience incorporates personal feelings as well as thoughts. Enabling people to express and manage emotions effectively can help to prevent stress-related illness, while addressing psychological as well as physical needs enhances patient satisfaction and may aid their recovery (Goleman, 2020). Goleman's book was inspired by research into emotional intelligence by Peter Salavoy and John Mayer. Since its publication there has been a growing recognition within healthcare education and corporate management training of the importance of becoming more self-aware and interpersonally skilled in this respect, such as learning how to both control and communicate feelings appropriately in one-to-one or group settings. In the case study, the Jewish nurse demonstrated that he had a high level of emotional intelligence in giving compassionate non-judgemental care to someone suspected of killing 11 Jews in the synagogue, who arrived in ER shouting 'Death to all Jews', and who reminded him of the racist abuse he had been a victim of in the past. It is remarkable that he was able to overcome the horror he felt at the mass killing targeting his faith in his local community, and his fear that his parents might have been victims, and that he too could be a target. Being able to control all of these feelings to avoid antagonising or escalating the hostile and threatening attitude of the patient/ prisoner appeared to have a calming influence as he thanked the nurse for treating his wounds. The nurse was also aware of the irony that the life of the suspected mass killer of Jews was, unbeknown to him, saved by a Jewish nurse, and the power of compassion over hatred and violence that this conveyed.

Activity 5.3   Stress management

The probability that events like those in the case study could happen to you is very unlikely, but it helps to highlight the importance of using emotional intelligence not just in caring for patients but also ourselves. As nurses, we are trained to be 'other regarding' and to develop therapeutic relationships in addressing their health problems. However, we also need to be 'engaged with self' to monitor and manage our own stress levels because if we don't look after our own mental health, we will be less effective or too burnt out to care for others.

To complete this activity, go to **www.nhs.uk/mental-health/self-help/guides-tools-and-activities/tips-to-reduce-stress/**. Here you will find an article entitled '10 stress busters' which gives advice about the best ways of dealing with stress. There are also links to further helpful information. Read through it and try applying one or two of the recommended ways to reduce stress. Reflect on whether this activity was useful or not and if you would recommend others to try it out for themselves.

As this activity is based on your own observations, there is no outline answer at the end of the chapter.

Developing and applying the 'other regarding' and 'engaged with self' dispositions of an evidence-based nurse go hand in hand because we use our self-agency in establishing caring relationships with others, and the feedback we receive from others can enhance our self-awareness and interpersonal skills. Indeed, 'connect with people' is one of the '10 stress busters' recommended in Activity 5.3 so that we can receive support when we need it to replenish our reserves and help us to support others more effectively. This is enabled through intersubjective understanding at a deeper level (not superficial 'chit chat') where there is mutual trust to communicate openly and honestly about things that matter to the people concerned. Our emotional intelligence (awareness, control, appropriate expression of our feelings plus empathising with others' feelings and responding appropriately) is developed through intersubjective understanding, and this enhances our sensitivity and ability to ensure that patients' preferences and needs are addressed in person-centred, evidence-based care.

Combining subjective–objective evidence-based nursing

As we embark on our careers in nursing and gradually make the transition from student to registered nurse, we are socialised through education, training and supervised clinical experience. In doing so, the personal knowledge we have accrued from subjective experience to date is continually supplemented by theoretical and practical knowledge from university and hospital or community practice placements. We are exposed to these influences in developing our professional identities as we learn to incorporate objective, critical thinking and reflexive skills alongside subjective, emotional intelligence and interpersonal skills. We can also find that the knowledge and skills we have acquired from previous life experiences are transferable to our current nursing roles, as the following case study helps to illustrate.

Case study: Sunitta's developing practice

Sunitta was in the first year of her nurse preparation programme and was trying to develop her practice. She had little experience in care settings, but came from a large extended family with whom she interacted a lot. Sunitta's practice supervisor was impressed with her ability to develop a therapeutic relationship with her patients. Sunitta would introduce herself and, with an easy manner, find out what they needed most. As she became more confident, Sunitta was able to deal with more challenging situations, such as working with a confused patient. However, Sunitta found it difficult to deconstruct what she did so fluently in practice in order to identify what it was that she did and ways of further improving it.

(Continued)

In order to provide evidence of how she was developing her practice of establishing therapeutic relationships, Sunitta needed to find a way to demonstrate how her practice was changing. Sunitta made use of a reflective approach that allowed her to use stories of her practice, which she then examined through reflective writing. Critically examining these stories in relation to communication theory helped Sunitta to develop her understanding of possible alternative strategies that she might use should the situation demand it. She also became clearer about how her communication responses were triggered and what she found difficult, which was a first step to being able to employ alternative strategies.

Discussing her practice experiences with others during an **action learning set** on her return to university helped Sunitta to identify some further ways of responding that some of her peers had used. One peer had needed to deal with conflict when a patient became very angry. Sunitta found this account especially helpful as she knew that conflict was something she avoided. She decided to return to the literature to find out more and to talk to her practice supervisor about this the next time she was in practice.

This case study illustrates personal as well as professional experiences in communication and relationship management (proficiency 4.3 – start of chapter) regarding subjective knowledge for practice. Personal and professional (theoretical and practical) knowledge interrelate and continue to develop and become transformed as they become integrated, informing each other and making something new. Nevertheless, it is also important to validate this knowledge. Sunitta did this by reading communication literature and through discussion with her practice supervisor. This is important in order to be able to articulate new knowledge.

You might find it easier to consider the development of self and the knowledge that you have as being like a giant jigsaw. You take all the experiences and understandings you have and try to create a giant picture of what you know; you do this by testing new experiences against what you know, or what you think you know. Sometimes you discard old knowledge or understandings, and sometimes you reject new knowledge and understandings; however, you can only safely do this by reflecting on experiences and testing them against other forms of understanding either alone (e.g. by reflection and seeking further information) or with others (e.g. in group discussion, teaching or action learning sets). However you proceed, you start to build up a picture of the world from your own point of view with your own understandings, and, as you become more questioning, you understand that there are bits of the picture missing; you use the influences on practice modified by the dispositions of an evidence-based nurse (Figure 1.1), which includes reflection, to continue to fill in these gaps, while understanding that the picture will never be finished.

There are various reflective models to guide your exploration of clinical experiences in order to relive and learn from them, and to develop both personally and professionally. They can help to put your personal, subjective thoughts and feelings into a wider context taking account of the views of patients, other parties involved and relevant theory or research. The What? So what? Now What? model (Driscoll, 2007) is the most straight-forward of these:

- **What?** – What happened? What was I thinking? What was I feeling? What did I do?
- **So what?** – What was the point? What did I achieve? Could I have achieved more?
- **Now what?** – What have I learned from this? What can I do differently next time?

Reflective practice can occur 'in-action' while carrying out our nursing duties or 'on-action' when looking back after the event to review what happened (Schön, 1983). In the next case study, the nurse is continually reflecting 'in-action' when sensing that something is not quite right with an unconscious patient (see NMC proficiency 1.17 at the start of chapter).

Case study: Detecting a case of tracheal stricture

Anja had been involved in a motorcycle accident while on holiday in Cyprus, where she had sustained extensive head injuries. These had left her in a **vegetative state**, although she was able to breathe on her own through a **tracheostomy tube** with supplementary oxygen. Anja had been transferred back to a hospital in the UK for assessment and the planning of her ongoing care. She was not suitable for admission to an intensive care unit or a high-dependency ward as her condition was categorised as chronic rather than acute, but Anja still required special nursing, particularly at night. Consequently, a number of flexi nurses were drafted in to help with her care.

During a night shift, Maureen – the nurse on duty – noticed that Anja seemed restless and 'just did not look right'. Anja's **vital signs** and **pulse oximetry** that Maureen recorded were within normal parameters for Anja, and there was no apparent incontinence or reason for discomfort as she was nursed on an airflow pressure mattress. Maureen decided to check the tracheostomy tube, first undertaking tracheal suction and then changing the tube, even though the pulse oximeter reading was normal. Anja remained restless.

Maureen was still not happy with Anja's condition, although she could not account for this. Maureen asked the anaesthetist to come and review Anja. The anaesthetist, who was relatively inexperienced, examined Anja and also could not find anything specific but called other medical colleagues for their opinion. By this stage, an hour had elapsed and Maureen noticed a sudden significant drop in Anja's pulse oximetry reading to well below the normal reading, which would, within the pulse oximetry guidelines, have signalled the need to call for medical assistance. By this time the medical consensus had already been reached to take Anja to theatre.

(Continued)

When Anja arrived in the anaesthetic room her respiration rate had climbed dramatically and she had emptied her bowels – another potential sign of stress. Anja was in theatre for some time where it was discovered that she had a 60 per cent stricture of her trachea (**tracheal stricture**). Because of the supplementary oxygen, this had not been reflected in the pulse oximetry recording, which measured the level of oxygen saturation of haemoglobin and not the effectiveness of pulmonary ventilation. Had Maureen relied only on the pulse oximeter readings to assess Anja's well-being, it might have taken longer for Anja to receive the medical intervention she needed. Maureen's experience had taught her to look at her patient as well as the physiological data, and to take note of her intuitive promptings.

We can use Driscoll's reflective framework to review Maureen's actions in the case study:

- **What?** Maureen sensed that there had been a deterioration in Anja's condition despite the fact that all of her vital signs appeared to be within the normal range and, apart from being a little restless, there were no other signs that she was distressed. As a precautionary measure, Maureen cleaned and changed the tracheostomy tube that Anja was breathing through, but this did not seem to make any difference. Maureen escalated her concerns by getting the anaesthetist to come and review Anja's condition, who did not find anything wrong but decided to ask medical colleagues for a second opinion. By this time Anja had deteriorated rapidly and was taken to theatre where they discovered her trachea (windpipe) had narrowed significantly, requiring surgical intervention to enable her to carry on breathing.
- **So what?** As an unconscious bedridden patient, Anja was particularly vulnerable and Maureen fulfilled her duty of care by trusting her intuition that something was wrong. By alerting the medical team about it, they were on hand to intervene quickly. If there had been a delay in taking Anja to theatre, her condition would have been even worse.
- **Now what?** Maureen learned that she could sense that something was wrong before it became obvious that this was the case. This validated her actions and encouraged her to trust and act on her intuition in future where this is called for.

The case study highlights the use of intuition, which is the most subjective form of human judgement as it relies on **tacit knowledge** and implicit understanding with which we get a feeling of what seems the right thing to do without being able to explain the reasons why. Benner's (1984) study of the development and progression of nursing knowledge identified intuitive knowing as an essential part of the advancing practice of the experienced nurse. This means that in complex situations the experienced nurse is able to identify solutions to problems that are difficult to explain but they know to be right – for example, dealing with emergencies or recognising unusual features within routine practice. Intuition and empathy form a part of such experiential and personal knowing that is not easily rationalised, more tentative and, therefore, uncertain (Thorne, 2020). Such abstractions have been called hunches, second nature, intelligent guesswork, unconscious competence, sixth sense, instinct or 'gut feeling' (Friedemann Smith et al., 2022). Given that the rationale for intuitive decisions cannot be articulated, we can only really justify our related actions if the outcome is successful, as it was in the case study. This highlights potential risks if we were to solely rely on intuition which turned out to be wrong. It is therefore important to use other more explicit problem-solving approaches alongside intuitive knowing in carrying out a precautionary risk assessment of proposed actions – for example, Maureen continued to observe Anja's vital signs and physiological data.

The case study reinforces the benefits of nurses integrating their subjective impressions with the available objective data to enhance patient care. Combining subjective knowledge of the person with the analysis of physiological data obtained (e.g. Anja's pulse oximetry readings and respiration rate) is an important part of nursing practice. The intersubjective element of this integration of knowledge is gained from seeing and examining the person/patient, as well as communicating with them and taking note of interactive information. It may seem a little strange or counter-intuitive to try to communicate with an unconscious patient, but it is good practice because it conveys respect for their humanity when attending to them. Research also indicates that talking to unconscious patients can have a stimulating effect, even if there are no obvious signs that anything has been registered. In a study of 60 unconscious patients, the use of daily structured communication messages was associated with improved levels of consciousness, decrease in physiological adverse events, lower behavioural pain scale scores, and shorter duration of mechanical ventilation/length of stay in ICU in the intervention group (Otham and El-hady, 2015). Consulting with colleagues concerning their professional opinion (as Maureen did with the anaesthetist and the anaesthetist did with medical colleagues) is another way of developing intersubjective understanding, which helps to inform collaborative team working and decision-making (see also Chapters 6 and 7).

Making sense of subjective experience is therefore an important part of developing as a nurse and in understanding what it means to *nurse*. Ultimately, all the theory and research that we are taught has to make sense to us as individuals in order for us to apply it as nurses. Learning a skill involves transforming explicit theoretical information into tacit **embodied knowledge**, which is manifested through intuitive and skilled action – what some call *craftsmanship* (Sennett, 2008). Similarly, learning the craft of compassionate nursing brings together theory, professional values, personal experiences, opportunities and motivations, such as curiosity in finding out more in order to do the best job you can for patients (Adamson, 2018). You will have noticed in life how some people are more curious than others and develop an understanding of various things, both professional and more day-to-day, not because they are particularly clever, but because they are inquisitive. In the sense discussed here, nurses need to both experience situations and be inquisitive enough to learn from them in order to develop their professional craftsmanship; it is not enough just to experience, you also need to question. This is why being questioning, reflective, reflexive, a critical thinker, a creative thinker and morally active are also identified as essential dispositions of an evidence-based nurse (Figure 1.1).

Applying reflexivity in reviewing subjective experience

Reflexivity means someone *being able to examine his or her own feelings, reactions, and motives (= reasons for acting) and how these influence what he or she does or thinks in a situation* (Cambridge, 2018). It therefore has similarities with reflection in reviewing subjective experience. The main difference between the two is that reflection focuses on understanding experiences we've had, whereas reflexivity focuses on understanding us, how we might have influenced the events, and whether we may have knowingly or unknowingly misrepresented what happened. Reflexivity is an important skill to develop in qualitative research which seeks to elicit and make sense of people's subjective experience. To access the data, qualitative researchers develop relationships with respondents, which raises questions about the authenticity of findings in representing their views as opposed to the researcher's. Qualitative researchers should spell out how they applied reflexivity in their reports and if you have to evaluate such reports, your criticism would be justified if this were not the case.

Reinharz (1997) developed a method to help researchers develop and review their reflexivity by identifying three categories of selves:

1. 'Brought selves' – past experience influencing us.
2. 'Research-based selves' – scientific methods influencing us.
3. 'Situationally created selves' – current experience influencing us.

Given that being reflexive was identified as one of the *dispositions of an evidence-based nurse* (Figure 1.1), it makes sense to try to apply Reinharz's 'three categories of selves' in nursing (Standing, 2020). Table 5.1 does so by matching them to nurses' personal (subjective), theoretical (objective) and practical experience (intersubjective), and identifies areas where reflexive awareness (objective–subjectivity) might enable professional growth.

Table 5.1 helps to illustrate the interplay between our personal, biographical, subjective experience accumulated thus far; theory input developing our objective logical, analytical skills; and practical experience developing our intersubjective understanding with patients and clinical colleagues. It also offers examples of reflexive awareness in relation to each of these areas, suggesting things we may need to learn in developing our professional identities.

	Experience to date	Reflexive awareness
Personal 'Brought selves' (subjective)	• Commitment to helping others • Relevant previous experience • Communication skills • Ability to take constructive criticism and learn from it	• May need to work on enabling people to help themselves • Cannot assume that there is nothing more to learn • Adapt for diverse population • May need to work on accepting positive feedback
Theoretical 'Research-based' selves (objective)	• Physical and social sciences • How to access and critically evaluate relevant information • How to use problem solving and reflective frameworks • Health and illness and ways that nurses make a difference	• Application to practice unclear • May need to work on developing this more analytical approach • May need to work on selecting the best one for the purpose • May need to overcome possible confusion about nurse's role
Practical 'Situationally created selves' (intersubjective)	• Contribute to clinical team • Supervised nursing practice • Experience helping patients • Apply theory to practice	• Unsure of role in the team • Nervous about being observed • Upset when a patient died • Did not set aside time to discuss

Table 5.1   Reflexive awareness in nursing applying Reinharz's three categories of selves

Activity 5.4   Reflexivity

Look again at Table 5.1 and decide whether you feel you can relate to the different 'selves', and the experiences and potential areas for reflexive awareness associated with them. Use the format to devise your own table and make any changes necessary for it to represent your experience of the different selves and your particular examples requiring reflexive awareness. Remember that reflexivity is about being open and honest with yourself about things that you need to learn or adapt in order to become a more effective nurse. In a sense, it is a way of looking after yourself by understanding your perceived needs in order to devise ways of addressing any gaps in knowledge/skills that helps you feel more confident and competent. It may also help to highlight other factors affecting your performance that you are not in a position to do anything about that may require organisational change. But you can still focus on those things that are within your gift to do something about in the meantime. This will also have a positive impact on your ability to understand, care for and relate to others, and on your ability to combine the different 'selves' in shaping your professional identity.

As this is based on your own reflections, there is no outline answer at the end of the chapter.

Reflexivity may also lead nurses to critically explore the organisations and structures within which they work and consider how they might contribute to more effective team-work and communication to enhance high-quality care and patient safety (McHugh et al., 2020). The critically **reflexive** practitioner utilises various strategies for developing knowledge, including engaging with their historical experience, reading and understanding literature, and reflecting on practice and social interaction. Literature can set the experience within a body of knowledge that might include research studies as well as other practitioner accounts that are instrumental in validating experience. Being reflexive involves focusing on opportunities for learning by interrogating subjective perceptions, and considering issues of power and how people are thought of or spoken about.

Critical reflexivity means considering what is being asked and how this might translate into personal practice and how this relates to the evidence available in different forms. This reflexive stance offers an opportunity to examine our assumptions and how we might be implicated in the structures we create in everyday working (Bolton and Delderfield, 2018). Making sense of subjective experience involves understanding how this has evolved over time, how it fits with the experiences of others, what the study of experiences has revealed and what actually happens in practice.

Healthcare is constantly changing, and as nurses we are faced with new knowledge every day. Responding reflexively to changes in knowledge involves being open to a range of positivist, naturalistic and interpretive paradigms, and critically reflecting on their relevance for our practice and how to apply this knowledge (Price, 2021). Such reflexive consideration may lead to new insights into assumptions about how knowledge is used and how practitioners may be instrumental in developing evidence through their reworking of knowledge. Hence, reflexive evaluation is an important method for transforming personal viewpoints and potential biases in positive ways (van Draanen, 2017).

Applying rigour in making sense of subjective experience

We have discussed the value of understanding our patients' subjective understanding in order to find out their thoughts, feelings and experiences about their situation, and preferred ways of dealing with it. We acknowledged the importance of delving into our own subjective experience, and through reflexive awareness identify the areas of personal and professional development we could work on to be better nurses. We also mentioned the impact of the social, environmental and organisational context in which care is delivered. In order to draw this together and summarise how we can authenticate and make sense of this array of subjective and intersubjective experience, it is worthwhile combining the criteria used by qualitative researchers. Table 5.2 provides a summary of these using the mnemonic FACTS.

F	**Fittingness**	How do findings appear to fit the social context they were derived from? Can learning be transferred to other contexts?
A	**Auditability**	How transparent, open to scrutiny by others is the audit trail in detailing each step of the process and evidence obtained?
C	**Credibility**	How much subjective adequacy of data is there? Would those whose experience is being reported recognise it as their own?
T	**Trustworthiness**	How was researcher reflexivity applied? How did respondents authenticate and validate the interpretations of the findings?
S	**Saturation**	Are the identified themes adequately supported by the findings? How are atypical/negative findings accounted for?

Table 5.2   FACTS mnemonic of rigour in making sense of subjective experience

Adapted from Hussein et al., 2015.

The FACTS criteria illustrate how it is possible to critique the way in which people's subjective experience has been presented and interpreted. Unlike quantitative research where the object is to eliminate subjectivity, in qualitative research the object is to capture authentic accounts of patients' and others' subjective experience, and make sense of them. You could also apply this framework to case studies, professional portfolios or other projects where the purpose is to obtain a more in-depth understanding of people's lived experience. In doing so, you will be helping to articulate the elusive subjective and intersubjective understanding that underpins nurses' professional knowledge and compassionate, empathetic and caring skills.

Chapter summary

This chapter has explored the concept of subjective experience, how to make sense of it, and how to apply it within the person-centred model of evidence-based practice in nursing described in Chapter 1. We noted that subjective experience relates closely to 'other regarding' and 'engaged with self' dispositions of an evidence-based nurse, and with 'experience' and 'patient preferences' influences on their practice. We discussed Erikson's theory of psychosocial development, emotional intelligence and how to deal with stress in the context of our individual and social identities and personal biographies. Case studies were used to illustrate the need to understand subjective experience in person-centred care with reference to NMC proficiencies. The importance of being reflexive was explored to minimise potential bias when eliciting or interpreting others' subjective understanding, and to highlight areas of personal, theoretical and practical knowledge where there is scope for development. We rounded things off by summarising FACTS qualitative criteria designed to ensure rigour and authenticity when making sense of subjective experience. It was recommended as a useful framework for readers in applying theory to practice.

Activities: Brief outline answers

Activity 5.2 Critical thinking (page 92)

1.   *What impact did caring for a suspected mass killer and hater of Jews have on the Jewish nurse?*

Horror at the tragic events, anxious about parents' safety, recall of racist bullying at school, conscious effort to show compassion for suspected killer as quiet statement against violence.

2.   *What impact did being cared for by the nurse appear to have on the suspected mass killer?*

He was admitted in an agitated and aggressive state shouting racist abuse, but appeared to calm down and express gratitude for life-saving help.

3.   *How did the nurse apply the 'dispositions of an evidence-based nurse' to practice?*

'Other regarding' – focused on treating the prisoner/patient's gunshot wounds, avoiding antagonising him, honouring victims of mass shooting. 'Engaged with self' – controlled feelings of fear or horror, appreciated the irony of Jewish nurse helping suspected mass killer of Jews.

4.   *Which 'influences on practice' provided evidence to support the nurse's actions?*

'Research evidence' concerning normal range of physiological observations; 'practice knowledge' in applying compression to stop bleeding; 'experience' as ER nurse dealing with acute emergencies; 'policy' guidelines governing clinical procedures; 'Resources' availability of theatre for surgical intervention; 'patient preference' avoided mentioning Jewish heritage given the prisoner/patient's anti-Semitic verbal abuse and being suspected of extreme violence and a horrific hate crime; 'views of other professionals' speedy hospital transfer by paramedics with police escort, surgical team on hand to repair gunshot wounds, Director of hospital briefed news channels about events; 'ethics' treated prisoner humanely and effectively despite his alleged crimes; 'law' police presence at all times to contain threat of further violence.

5.   *How effectively were the principles of person-centred care applied to practice?*

The prisoner/patient was provided with the emergency life-saving care he required to survive multiple gunshot wounds. The extensive injuries and his initial threatening demeanour meant that shared decision-making was not really an option. The nurse felt that he offered kindness and compassion, which seems to be borne out when the prisoner/patient thanked him for care.

6.   *How might the nurse's biography/psychosocial development have influenced his career choice?*

The abusive racist intimidation and bullying experienced by the nurse at school would probably have affected his sense of belonging and security. In resolving the psychosocial identity versus role confusion crisis, he opted not to follow his father in becoming a rabbi, but chose an alternative form of public service. In resolving the intimacy versus isolation crisis, the nurse has found a way of being socially accepted where he can apply his caring nature.

Further reading

Barker, S (2016) *Psychology for Nurses and Healthcare Professionals: Developing Compassionate Care.* London: Sage.

Explains a range of psychological approaches in delivering compassionate care.

Price, B (2022) *Delivering Person-Centred Care in Nursing.* London: Learning Matters/Sage.

Discusses principles of person-centred care, then demonstrates its many applications.

Useful websites

www.patientstories.org.uk

Access to information and films documenting the poignant stories that patients and relatives have to tell about their experiences of healthcare.

www.simplypsychology.org

Access to a wide variety of informative psychology articles and learning materials. Scroll down to A–Z index and pick a topic – e.g., Erikson's psychosocial theory.

Chapter 6

Working with others to achieve evidence-based care

Peter Ellis

Chapter aims

After reading this chapter, you will be able to:

- describe why working with others in the planning of evidence-based care is important;
- identify the different groups of individuals it is important to work with to achieve evidenced care;
- demonstrate awareness of some of the barriers to interprofessional evidence-based care delivery;
- understand why service users' views are important in the delivery of evidence-based nursing practice.

Introduction

So far in this book we have explored some of the skills you need to work as an individual nurse providing evidence-based nursing care. We have identified some challenges that might face the nurse who is attempting to provide evidence-based care and have presented some tools for you to use for yourself when developing as an evidential nurse ready for the challenges of lifelong learning.

Nursing care does not take place in a vacuum. The complexities of modern care mean that there is a need for any number of formal and informal care givers to provide the care that any individual patient needs. There are also care delivery issues that need to be accounted for, such as the experience of care and the individual needs and wishes of each patient.

This chapter will present an overview of some of the issues that face nurses when working with others, including patients. It will also present an argument, first described in Chapter 1, that working effectively with others is a necessary part of the delivery of evidence-based nursing care. As with the rest of the book, the issues here are that no single element of care can be considered on its own and that no one element of the caring process takes precedence over another. Rather, the argument about evidence-based care presented in this book frames evidence-based nursing as the delivery of holistic, multifaceted and multiprofessional care, which is supported by lifelong learning, ethical sensitivity and moral activity, reflection and reflexivity as well as an understanding of research, experiential elements of learning and, above all, the needs and wishes of the individual patient.

It is clear that the argument made here is quite complex. It is an argument that responds to some of the greyness existing at the boundaries of theory and practice, and, it is hoped, prepares or further develops the ability of nurses to advance the quality of their practice in a meaningful, considered and patient-focused manner where they act as a professional role model.

This chapter illuminates some of the elements of Figure 1.1 ('The influences on and dispositions of an evidence-based nurse'; see p24) in which we saw that delivering patient-centred care requires multiple strands of conscious decision-making to run simultaneously. We saw how various dispositions (or elements of our character) affect the ways in which we can engage as evidential, patient-centred practitioners. One of these dispositions, which is an important aspect of the current chapter, is to be 'other regarding'.

Furthermore, we saw in the 'influences on practice' that there is a role for 'patient preference' as well as the 'views of other professionals'. What they amount to is the need to manage personal choices and behaviours, as well as seeking and nurturing interpersonal relationships, which, with resolve and some practice, enable nurses to deliver care in a manner that is both evidence-driven and patient-centred. This chapter is about exploring the interpersonal relationship aspect of this evidence-based nursing practice.

Service users' views

Taking account of the views of services users, the patient's voice, is high on the governmental agenda (DH, 2000, 2010, 2012b). This agenda is clearly reflected in the Standards of Proficiency for Registered Nurses by the Nursing and Midwifery Council (NMC, 2018a), some of which are highlighted at the start of the chapter.

What, then, is a service user? Service users fall into one of two categories: those who are current users of caring services such as health and social care, and those who are potential future users of these same services. This explains why the term 'patient' is not used consistently throughout this chapter. In fact, we are all actual and potential users of health and social care (Connelly and Seden, 2003), but most of the time we are not patients and would not necessarily like to be thought of as such. Most of us have accessed care on a number of occasions in our lives, be that because we are ill or because we are being screened for disease or vaccinated against some communicable disease.

Some consumers of care are residents in nursing and care homes, and are in receipt of social, perhaps more than health, care as such, but are still, broadly speaking, service users. The need for evidential care is as great in these settings as it is anywhere else, including community settings and in people's own homes. The reader is reminded therefore to consider the full breadth and depth of nursing when considering what it means to work with others in the delivery of care.

What, then, is important about the views of services users about the delivery of care? Clearly, most service users have a limited amount of knowledge about the hard science of care delivery and may not have a view about the quality of X-ray services, the choice of wound dressing used in the hospital or the biochemistry services' use of particular assays. What they – and we – do have, however, is significant experience of how we like to be treated in the care environment, and how we experience both illness and care. We all also have our own views about the extent of the care that we may wish to receive and how this affects us as individuals. In this respect, service users' views reflect the service element of the care they receive, much in the same way they may rate telephone appointments or the long waiting lists for care which are the legacy of COVID-19.

Activity 6.1   Reflection

Consider the last time you used a healthcare facility or had a telephone consultation. What were the positive elements of the experience? What were the negative elements of the experience? Thinking about your interactions, what, if anything, will you change about how you interact with service users? Has your thinking about communication in care settings been changed by your experiences during the pandemic?

As this activity is based on your own reflection, there is no outline answer at the end of the chapter.

Clearly, as well as the human elements of taking account of people's views about their own care, there are several moral and ethical imperatives that we, as nurses, must take account of in the delivery of care (Ellis, 2020). Perhaps the most important ethical principle, as it applies to this section of the book, is the imperative to respect the autonomy of individuals.

Autonomy is about the freedom to choose. In part, the process of consent supports this freedom of choice and involves the nurse who is delivering care in ensuring that the recipient of care understands what might happen to them (information giving and individual competence), is free from coercion (undue pressure) and understands what the alternative forms of care are – if there are any (Beauchamp and Childress, 2013). The final element of autonomy is the freedom to choose: people who have had the information given and understand it and who are free from coercion, have the right to decide whether to take the advice of the care giver or not. In fact, under the Mental Capacity Act (Her Majesty's Government, 2005) people have the right to make choices about their care which may appear to professionals to be bad choices, so long as they have the capacity (ability) to do so.

Issues of both advocacy and empowerment are important to the evidence-based nurse who is focused on delivering high-quality care that is based on evaluated knowledge and is what the service user actually wants. Some definitions regard advocacy as simply the process of representing the views of someone to someone else – for example, Dubler (1992, p85) defines advocacy within the caring professions as *acting to the limit of professional ability to provide for the client's interests and needs as the patient defines them.*

In Dubler's view, then, an advocate puts to one side their own view of a situation and represents only the point of view of the person they are advocating for. This view of advocacy actually represents the true meaning of the word quite well, as it stresses the importance of only representing the views of the client and no one else. This simple view of advocacy falls a little short of the realities of nursing care, though, in that it makes assumptions about the capacity (mental competence) and understanding of the facts by the individual client. It also misses the point where the decision is tainted by misapprehension or negative prior experiences.

Within this book, advocacy as it applies to the evidence-based nurse is a term used to define a process of representing the views of a service user when the nurse has ensured that they have discussed the nature of the intervention with the service user and have highlighted the alternatives available and the evidence for each potential course of action. Furthermore, the morally active evidence-based nurse will also ensure that the service user has understood what has been said, and that they are able and free to make a rational choice about what they want to happen.

Empowerment and advocacy in this respect are seen as different stages along the same continuum of service-user-focused care, with empowerment defined as enabling service users to become active participants, partners, in their care (Weisbeck et al., 2019). As in the definition of advocacy, the service user must be in receipt of the information they need to make their decision and they must understand the information. This definition of empowerment, like that of advocacy, recognises that the majority of people are able and willing to engage in decision-making about their own care. Both definitions further recognise that this is the service user's right and that some people will choose to exercise it and others will not or, indeed, cannot. Notably, nurses acting to empower or advocate for patients may find themselves in conflict with other professionals (Anantapong et al., 2021), so taking on this role requires courage.

That said, some service users will make the choice not to engage with decision-making, and perhaps even not to hear what the professionals have to say about their care options. This can also be considered to represent the exercise of autonomy for these individuals and should not be ignored.

Activity 6.2   Reflection

Return to the model of evidence-based nursing presented in Chapter 1 (see Figure 1.1 on p24) and reflect on the nature of the process of decision-making discussed there. Identify especially the ethical elements of the model and the elements that apply to decision-making that take into account service user preferences and the dispositions of the evidence-based nurse that are 'other regarding'. How do you see these as contributing to user consultation as highlighted in this section?

An outline answer is provided at the end of the chapter.

Service users' views also extend to understanding the views of individuals – and groups of individuals – who are not currently in receipt of care. These views help to shape our understanding of the context within which care is received and therefore how it might best be delivered.

On a macro level, these views are sought through governmental and local authority consultation, while more disease-specific groups might be a source of understanding and knowledge about specific elements of care services delivery. The NHS run consultations with service users more or less constantly – e.g., via engage.england.nhs.uk. In these, they seek the opinions of 'NHS staff, patients, stakeholders and the public' in their quest to improve health outcomes. The Cancer Partnership Project – a joint venture between Macmillan Cancer Relief and the Department of Health that consulted widely among professionals and cancer sufferers on the provision and delivery of cancer services – was regarded as a successful model of consultation and led to effective changes in cancer care provision in the UK (Sitzia et al., 2004).

More locally, patient groups, such as hospital-affiliated kidney or cardiac patients' associations, play a useful role in identifying areas of concern for patients and care providers, as well as in supporting changes to care delivery. One of the key lines of enquiry (the so-called KLOEs) for the domain 'responsive' inspected under the current Care Quality Commission (CQC) regimen in nursing and care homes looks to see if the registered manager consults with residents and families about their care by, for example, undertaking satisfaction surveys, collecting comments and having house meetings.

What is evident is that a move away from professional-driven care has occurred in the UK and that the voice of patients, or service users, is increasingly being heard, although this may have been paused somewhat during the COVID-19 pandemic.

Activity 6.3   Research and finding out

Go online to the **gov.uk** website and find the pages for the Department of Health and Social Care. Once on these pages, find the current consultations that are underway – look under policy papers and consultations. Spend some time looking at the characteristics of the consultations and considering their nature and diversity; consider which ones apply to people currently in the receipt of care and which ones do not. Think about why this might be and consider which ones you might usefully contribute to.

As this activity is based on your own reflection, there is no outline answer at the end of the chapter.

Evidence operates at two levels. At the first level, it provides evidence for care in its own right – that is to say, the experience of the service user, the *symptoms* they express and their interpretation of the care they receive provide evidence for nursing. For example, only the service user can know if they feel pain, are upset or anxious – remember as nurses we cannot directly measure symptoms, we can only see and measure signs of illness and disease. We cannot validate these symptoms through direct objective mechanisms as we have no machine to measure pain or anxiety as such. We can, however, use some objective measures to validate what they are telling us, such as noting a rise in blood pressure or that the patient is sweating, crying or perhaps trembling. We can also validate what the service user is telling us about what they feel through our own subjective interpretation and understanding of what they are experiencing on a human level – through common understanding of human experience, what might be called **intersubjectivity**.

At the second level, subjective evidence might serve to validate observations that we have made for ourselves using more objective measures. For example, if we take a blood sugar reading for a service user with diabetes and find that they are hypoglycaemic (have a low blood sugar level), we might expect them to tell us that they feel tired, hungry or confused.

What these examples show is that in our day-to-day practice we see interplay between what we can measure and observe for ourselves and what the service user tells us. The argument here is that whichever way round the information comes to us – service users telling us their symptoms or us observing signs – as nurses we are often alert to, and able to handle, the interplay between more than one source of evidence for practice at any one time. In *Understanding Research for Nursing Students* (also in this series), Chapter 6 discusses in detail the concept of triangulation which is about validating information using more than one information source.

Sometimes evidence can be contradictory: the service user tells us they are not in pain, but we observe them wincing or gritting their teeth. On such occasions it is communication that helps us to express our concerns to the service user and demonstrate both our disposition to be 'other regarding' and the advancing influence of increasing 'practice knowledge' (see Figure 1.1 on p24). Evidently, in this scenario there is also a need to exercise the disposition of being both 'ethically sensitive' and 'morally active' in seeking via good communication to act in what will be in the best interests of our patient.

What seems clear is that whatever we think about the motivations behind the advance of the evidence-based practice agenda, as nurses we practise it daily within our working lives. Perhaps awaking our understanding of what evidence-based practice means for nursing on a more macro scale requires that we become more aware of how the principles of evidence-based nursing practice operate at this micro level to inform our day-to-day practice.

In this section, we have identified that user consultation is an important element of the government's agenda and that it is identified by the NMC as a required competency for all nurses. We have seen that there is a moral imperative for the evidence-based nurse to take into account service users' views, and that advocacy and empowerment are key strategies for making this a reality of the care process. We have also seen how interaction and exploration of subjectivity enable the nurse operating on a day-to-day basis to be evidence-based in their care provision and that understanding how this operates might help us to understand the importance of evidence-based practice for nursing on a much broader scale.

Before we go on to explore further strategies for identifying service users' views, it is important that we identify some of the barriers to consultation that might impact on the evidence-based nurse.

Barriers to service user consultation

By understanding the potential problems, we are better able to understand how something might be made to work better. We have identified that user consultation takes place at two key levels: at the one-to-one level, where the concern is the care of an individual; and at the group level, where the concern is the general care provided to a group of service users. We will examine some of the barriers to effective consultation at each of these levels.

Communication and interaction with service users are the cornerstone of good nursing care. Communication is time-consuming, however, and the sharing of information and ensuring that information is understood can take precious time out of the nurse's day. Information sharing and frank and open discussion are not easy to undertake in the ward environment where there are distractions and the very real possibility that a consultation will be overheard by others. Our own lack of knowledge and a fear of demonstrating this to patients may make some nurses feel uncomfortable about discussing options for care.

As well as physical and personal barriers to communication and consultation, there are barriers that are created because of the position we hold, or feel we hold, in the multidisciplinary team. This may lead some nurses to be coy about discussing the possibilities of care with patients because they feel that ultimately someone else will make the decision about care. At other times, we may feel unable to put into language that the service user will understand the various options for their care. We may feel we are best placed to make a decision about the care of service users, especially where individual service users appear less than able to make such decisions for themselves – as might be the case for some adults with learning difficulties.

It is situations like these that highlight the very real need for morality and ethics to feature strongly in any framework of evidence-based nursing. It would be easier to operate in a moral vacuum where we make choices for our service users based on what we think are in their medical (or nursing) best interests (Ellis, 2019). However, such an understanding of evidence-based care misses the point that 'best interests' not only include physical elements, but also psychosocial values and beliefs as well as life experiences that make us all unique as human beings (NICE, 2020). This highlights the need not only for a subjective and intersubjective interpretation of evidence, but also for good communication and a commitment to morally active nursing, advocacy and empowerment.

Service users themselves may present a number of difficulties for the nurse trying to discuss care options. The vulnerability that may arise out of illness, physical or mental disability, age or language can stand in the way of effective two-way communication.

Activity 6.4   Critical Thinking

Many people have chosen not to have any of the vaccinations against COVID-19. It may be that you have met such people who have become unwell as a result. Who or what might have influenced their decision? What form of best interests do you think are enacted in such situations?

As this activity is based on your own critical thinking, there is no outline answer at the end of the chapter.

Other barriers to good communication and taking account of the opinions and experiences of service users include our own orientations to other people and the beliefs we hold about the value of this sort of interaction. Sometimes we make assumptions about what service users do and do not know because they are not care professionals like us or, indeed, because they come from a caring background and therefore we feel they should know about their own care needs. At other times, we make the assumption that because they have been seen by another member of the team, they have all the information they need and we do not need to engage with them because they do not need to hear the information twice or because it is hard for us to have difficult conversations.

On many occasions, we feel too self-conscious to explore the service user's opinions about their care because their condition is too embarrassing to talk about or we feel out of our depth discussing issues such as death or mental illness. Sometimes the service users' wishes, opinions and experiences take us out of our comfort zones.

So, how might we function in such scenarios and how might we develop the characteristics and dispositions of the morally active evidence-based nurse?

Activity 6.5   Reflection

Think about the last time you did not share difficult information with a service user or family member. What was going on in your mind that stopped you from having the conversation? Were you scared about their potential response? Why could you not manage to find the right words to say? What was the result of you not having the conversation for the service user and their family?

As this activity is based on your own reflection, there is no outline answer at the end of the chapter.

Working effectively with service users

In order to overcome the difficulties and barriers that stop us communicating well with service users, we have to take the initiative. It is not really possible to be an ethically sensitive or morally active evidence-based nurse without communicating with service users about their experiences and engaging them in the planning of their own care. At a one-to-one level, there are a number of strategies we can employ that will make this role easier and allow us to add being 'other regarding' and 'engaged with self' to our list of personal qualities.

Overcoming barriers to communication as a student or junior nurse requires us to make time to spend constructively with our service users and to use this time wisely. Clearly, the personal barriers to communication are ours to overcome. Investing time in reflection, either singly or in a group, is a useful strategy in allowing us to identify these barriers and ways in which they might be overcome (Jasper, 2013). Some strategies towards achieving good communication are presented in Table 6.1.

- Practise – go out of your way to communicate with service users, especially when the subject matter is difficult.
- Try to find somewhere private to talk.
- Choose an appropriate time to engage in talk and ensure that the service user knows how long you might have.
- Get yourself a chair and sit at eye level with the service user; this demonstrates that you have time and brings you down to their physical level.
- Speak clearly, avoiding medical jargon and the use of metaphors.
- If you are giving information, concentrate only on key messages.
- Repeat the key messages.
- Ask the service user to recap to you their understanding of the information.
- Supplement information giving with leaflets, pictures and models; if these are not available, write your own notes for the service user.
- Paraphrase to check what you hear the service user saying: 'Are you saying that . . . ?'
- Encourage questions; do not say 'Have you any questions?'; instead try 'What questions have you got?'

Table 6.1   Some strategies for achieving good communication

While developing these communication skills, it is useful to reflect on how an interaction went – either alone (perhaps using a reflective diary) or with other people. Of course, the important element of this reflection process is learning from what went well and what did not go so well in order to plan your approach to communicating in the future.

It may seem odd that we concentrate on good communication in a book about evidence-based practice, but there are many benefits that accrue from good communication for both evidence-based nursing and the nurse–service user relationship. Some of these benefits are identified in Table 6.2.

From the point of view of the evidence base of nursing, communication is an absolute necessity. It is the service user who knows not only how they feel physically, but also how they feel about their experience of care. Without interacting with the service user, we cannot know if what we do as nurses is effective, nor can we know if what we do is appreciated and if the experience of care is good.

- An understanding of what is going on can mean that the service user experiences less pain and fewer other symptoms (Hayward, 1979).
- Satisfaction with care can be increased (Ali, 2017).
- Positive patient outcomes is promoted (Afriyie, 2020).
- Good communication demonstrates that the nurse is person-centred.
- Subjective data can be collected and used to inform the planning of the service user's care.
- Patients have the information they need to make informed decisions.

Table 6.2   Some of the benefits of good communication

Working with other professionals

One of the influences on practice that we identified in our model of evidence-based nursing in Chapter 1 was 'views of other professionals'. As we saw in Chapter 5, an understanding and interpretation of the subjective views of others can add greatly to both the amount of knowledge we have and also its depth. Working with other professionals is often termed collaborative practice or interprofessional working, and implies something more than the traditional notion of multidisciplinary working that may be regarded as less integrated, although the real proof of the level of integration lies in the way in which joint working is undertaken and not in the name.

At its simplest, collaboration is about working together, which implies a commonality of purpose but not a unification of being; it comprises conscious interactions between individuals in order to achieve shared goals by the overlapping of activities rather than merely working alongside colleagues (Meads et al., 2005). Similarly, interprofessional working has been defined as different healthcare professionals interacting together *productively to provide high-quality patient care* (Yoost and Crawford, 2022). As such, interprofessional working is seen as being much broader in its scope than multidisciplinary teamwork and is not just about how practitioners work together, but rather about how they manage and plan tasks for the benefit of service users, groups or services.

Within the context of this book, therefore, interprofessional working and collaboration are more about who the individual is rather than what they do – it is one of the dispositions identified in Chapter 1 as being 'other regarding', which supports the notion of allowing the views of other professionals to influence nursing practice. What is important here for the student nurse is that you develop a way of being and of practising nursing which is permanently tuned into the benefits of interprofessional working and the benefits this brings to the service user; it really is not just enough to know about interprofessionality, it is necessary to feel it and allow it to become one of our character traits, our dispositions.

So what are the benefits of interprofessional practice and collaboration for the evidence-based nurse? In their Cochrane review of the evidence for interprofessional collaboration, Reeves et al. (2017) identified that evidence for its benefits remains poor, but conclude that this is due to difficulties encountered in clinical practice and that further research is needed.

In the scheme that was presented in Chapter 1, evidence-based nursing is seen as the ability to think judiciously about different strands of information that may collectively be drawn together to create evidence. We saw in Chapter 5 that some of the influences on practice include subjective information and the ability to assimilate this into our understanding of the delivery of care through reflection and reflexivity.

Put simply, the point is this: if we are happy to allow our own experience and reflections to guide the care that we give, then it is perhaps egocentric not to afford this same level of respect to the experiences and reflections of others. There are two good reasons for respecting the experiences and reflections of others: first, we ourselves cannot have experience of everything; second, some individuals have trained in specialist and different areas of care than we, as nurses, have, and this may mean their understandings of and reflections on care may be more sophisticated and better informed than ours.

This notion of being aware of and open to the knowledge that exists within other professions reflects the nature of nursing, which is essentially an eclectic and holistic application of knowledge that we have gained, and honed, from other disciplines. Put simply, by choosing to listen to and work cooperatively with other professionals, we grow as practitioners and the care we can give service users improves.

There is, of course, a caveat to this acceptance of what others tell us: it must make sense. Like all information accepted as knowledge used to inform the individual evidence base, it is important that we subject it to some scrutiny for ourselves. This is the critical thinking that is alluded to in Chapter 1 and that is discussed again in Chapter 8. This idea of checking also reflects one of the messages in Chapter 5 and earlier in this chapter – that we can use subjective knowledge to validate other subjective knowledge (perhaps other people's views on something we also have a view on) or even to validate more objective forms of knowledge such as the findings of research.

Activity 6.6   Communication

Next time you have the opportunity to work with a professional from a different background in the delivery of care, ask them this simple question: 'What are your priorities for the care of this individual and why are these important to you?' Then take some time to reflect on what this means for you as a nurse and how what they said contributes to what it is that you are trying to achieve for the service user – or not.

An outline answer is provided at the end of the chapter.

In essence, then, failing to account for the experience and knowledge of our professional colleagues shuts the door to a very important avenue of learning, which in turn impacts on our ability to develop a holistic evidence base both individually for the service user in front of us now and more generally in the creation of our own bank of professional knowledge.

As with the intersubjectivity and understanding about the service users' experience of pain, which we discussed earlier, working with colleagues from different disciplines allows us to both validate and to ask questions about our developed, and developing, understanding of care. Quite simply, and returning to the earlier observation that nursing does not take place in a vacuum, working in a meaningful way with professional colleagues, and informal carers, allows us to both understand and offer a richer and more meaningful experience of care to service users – something we deny them if we choose to work alone.

As well as the concept of learning from professionals from other backgrounds, as nurses we need to continue to learn from each other. The same arguments about why this is important and the need to be critical in our adoption of new knowledge apply here as in the examples of adopting evidence from other professionals.

Barriers to working with other professionals

There are a number of issues that act as barriers to interprofessional collaboration and therefore by default to the development of our own holistic evidence base. These barriers – some of which relate to how we see ourselves as individuals and as nurses and some of which arise as a result of the way in which care is organised – need to be understood before they can be overcome.

We said in Figure 1.1 (p24) that being 'engaged with self' is an important attribute of the evidence-based nurse. But what does this mean?

Being engaged with self is not only about understanding who we are and where we have come from both personally and professionally, but also about understanding our motivations, understandings, biases and prejudices. This is not merely about cultural, racial, gender or disability stereotyping; it is about our disposition towards others. Are we willing to engage with others, learn from others, and adapt not only our knowledge but perhaps even our values as a result of these interactions? Or are we unable to see the points of view or the understandings that others have and use these to inform not only what we know but perhaps even who we are?

The NMC Standards of Proficiency for Registered Nurses require that we *must work with people, their families, carers and colleagues to develop effective improvement strategies for quality and safety, sharing feedback and learning from positive outcomes and experiences, mistakes and adverse outcomes and experiences* (NMC, 2018a, p23) and also that we must *have underpinning communication skills for assessing, planning, providing and managing best practice, evidence-based nursing care* (NMC, 2018a, p28).

The point quite simply is this: we cannot show integrity in our practice and in our communication with others, nor develop as evidential practitioners, unless we actually believe and adopt this value of interprofessional and collaborative practice for real. Integrity requires that this is not a charade, as integrity means acting and communicating in ways that we actually believe.

This does not mean that we should blindly accept what other people tell us or that we should allow service users to make what are essentially uninformed bad decisions about their care. The evidence-based morally active nurse takes account of many issues in generating a plan of care using both objective and subjective information.

As well as potential philosophical differences in our approaches to care, other barriers can stand in the way of good collaborative interprofessional care, as shown in Table 6.3. The existence of barriers to interprofessional working, and failure to act because we think others are, have given rise to a number of tragedies over the years, including the deaths of Victoria Climbié in 2000 (Laming, 2003), Baby P in 2007 (Care Quality Commission, 2009) as well as Daniel Pelka in 2012 (Rogers, 2013). Clearly, there are negative consequences of not working in interprofessional ways that extend beyond not creating and operating within a holistic evidence base.

- Professional rivalries
- Poor understanding of each other's terminology
- Lack of trust
- Professional labelling and stereotyping
- Traditional hierarchies of care
- Unrealistic expectations
- Lack of resources and management support

Table 6.3   Some barriers to interprofessional working

Based on the work of Barber et al. (2009).

Strategies for working with other professionals

How, then, can we get to a point at which we work in a more integrated manner with other professionals? What benefits accrue for evidence-based nursing practice if we do? The first of these questions is hard to answer because alone we are unlikely to change ways of working, although we can certainly be role models of collaborative practice. Perhaps by answering the second question – what benefits accrue and for whom? – will enable us to return to the first question and answer it in a meaningful way.

The benefits of collaborative working – certainly within the scheme of evidence-based practice that we are exploring in this book – arise out of the improved ability to deliver person-centred holistic care. Consider Activity 6.7.

Activity 6.7   Critical thinking

John is a 72-year-old man who is admitted to the nursing home in which you are undertaking a placement. John has insulin-dependent diabetes and, as a result, has a diabetic foot ulcer, retinopathy and moderate chronic kidney disease. John is quite frail and requires help with many of the activities of daily living.

Given John's multiple and varied needs, list all the staff groups who might need to be involved in his care, and state why.

An outline answer is provided at the end of the chapter.

What is clear from the answer to Activity 6.7 is that John will benefit from the input of many different professional groups from within the home and potentially from those outside the home. The benefit that interprofessional working brings to John's care, assuming the nursing home nurse co-ordinates his care, is that John receives appropriate and informed care and advice from the person most able to provide it. His care is the best it can be, and all the professionals involved contribute to this. At the centre of this care is John, who is supported by his named nurse. This nurse co-ordinates not only who sees John but also, more importantly, the delivery of the care that is advised, not for him so much as in collaboration with him. Everyone benefits, there is reduced duplication of effort and John gets the care he needs.

How can we as nurses achieve this? Certainly in Activity 6.7 none of this would be possible if the nurse involved was not alert to the possibilities that interprofessional working affords. By role modelling good interprofessional practice, the nurse is able to receive information from each of the care professionals involved and use this to plan John's care with him. This receptiveness to the input of other professionals is not received blindly; questions are asked, and the ideas and input received are tested against the nurse's existing understanding and knowledge.

Chapter summary

This chapter has expanded on the nature and purpose of working in an integrated manner with others, including service users, to achieve good-quality, evidential care. We have seen that there are a number of barriers to working with others, some of which are created by us and some of which are the result of human nature. We have further identified some important strategies for overcoming these barriers and some good ethical reasons why we must.

Consultation with service users has been framed as a means of improving not only what we do, but also the way that we do it. We have identified that such consultation is, in reality, the only means we have by which we can understand the way in which care is experienced. We have explored to some extent the need for interprofessional working to achieve high-quality service user care given that the care needs of individuals are increasingly complex. We have seen that evidence-based practice requires a service-user-focused (person/patient-centred) approach to care and must be ethical, responding to and overcoming the potential difficulties this poses.

In this chapter there are clearly a number of very big challenges that the busy nurse must face and overcome if they are to achieve care that is responsive to the requirements of the government, the NMC, the research evidence and, most importantly, the service users who we are here to serve.

Activities: Brief outline answers

Activity 6.2 Reflection (page 110)

Being mindful of the opinions, experiences and beliefs of others is a fundamental aspect of moral and ethical behaviour when applied to the process of drawing on evidence to inform nursing practice. Throughout the book, we have seen that the evidence base for nursing is not merely about what we do, but also about how we go about our work – how it is experienced by others. Within the model of evidence-based nursing there is a need to acknowledge that not everything we do has a basis in scientific or research-based knowledge and that some of the sources of knowledge we use draw upon the experiences and understandings of others. To achieve these lofty goals, the nurse therefore needs to be mindful of others while creating for themselves an evidence base in which their practice can be safely and ethically grounded.

Activity 6.6 Communication (page 118)

Nursing goals are often quite broad and represent an attempt to attend to the holistic care of an individual service user. Within these holistic goals will invariably sit a number of single and discrete goals that are shared by other care professionals. For example, the occupational therapist may aim to restore the ability to self-care, while the physiotherapist may regard their chief aim as enabling the service user to mobilise safely. Both of these examples reflect the overall aims of nursing, which often relate to enabling the service user to achieve self-care safely. On a broader view, all three approaches are about contributing to care. If we look at the subjective validity of these three views on care, we can see that there is a fair degree of overlap, which helps to validate the three different, but converging viewpoints.

Activity 6.7 Critical thinking (page 120)

John might benefit from seeing the following specialist staff:

- The specialist nurses and doctors of the diabetes team would help him get better control of his diabetes.
- The tissue viability nurse might provide valuable insights into managing John's ulcer.
- The ophthalmologist would prove useful in managing John's deteriorating vision.
- The nephrology consultant would be able to make informed decisions with John relating to his kidney disease.
- The dietitian might help John with both his renal and diabetic diet.
- The pharmacist would be useful in helping to rationalise John's medication.
- The nursing home nurses and healthcare support workers will be able to identify a plan of care for John such that his activities of daily living needs are properly met.
- John's social worker/care manager could help John apply for appropriate welfare benefits.
- The occupational therapist could help John adapt his home to accommodate his deteriorating vision.

The home's activities team will be able to help John find things to do to occupy his time and to stimulate him while the kitchen staff will provide the diet identified by the dietitian.

Further reading

Ellis, P (2022) *Understanding Research for Nursing Students* (3rd edn). London: Sage.

See Chapter 6 to gain a better understanding of triangulating data.

Goodman, B and Clemow, R (2010) *Nursing and Collaborative Practice* (2nd edn). Exeter: Learning Matters.

Contains a great deal of material and activities pertinent to working with others.

Koubel, G and Bungay, H (eds) (2009) *The Challenge of Person-Centred Care: An Interprofessional Perspective.* Basingstoke: Palgrave.

A comprehensive look at the patient as the centre of the care process.

Koubel, G and Bungay, H (eds) (2012) *Rights, Risks and Responsibilities: Interprofessional Perspectives.* Basingstoke: Palgrave.

See Chapter 1 for some ideas about what best interests might mean and Chapter 10 about responsibilities when working interprofessionally.

Thomas, J, Pollard, KC and Sellman, D (eds) (2014) *Interprofessional Working in Health and Social Care: Professional Perspectives* (2nd edn). London: Palgrave.

See especially Chapter 3 for working with service users.

Useful websites

www.caipe.org.uk

Website of the Centre for the Advancement of Interprofessional Education.

www.tandfonline.com/toc/ijic20/current

Link to the *Journal of Interprofessional Care*.

https://valuesbasedpractice.org/

Website of the Collaborating Centre for Values-based practice in Health and Social Care.

Chapter 7

Clinical decision-making in evidence-based nursing

Mooi Standing

NMC Future Nurse: Standards of Proficiency for Registered Nurses

This chapter will address the following platforms and proficiencies:

Platform 1: Being an accountable professional

At the point of registration, the registered nurse will be able to:

1.9   understand the need to base all decisions regarding care and interventions on people's needs and preferences, recognising and addressing any personal and external factors that may unduly influence their decisions.

Platform 2: Promoting health and preventing ill health

At the point of registration, the registered nurse will be able to:

2.10   provide information in accessible ways to help people understand and make decisions about their health, life choices, illness and care.

Platform 3: Assessing needs and planning care

At the point of registration, the registered nurse will be able to:

3.6   effectively assess a person's capacity to make decisions about their own care and to give or withhold consent.

Platform 4: Providing and evaluating care

At the point of registration, the registered nurse will be able to:

4.2   work in partnership with people to encourage shared decision making in order to support individuals, their families and carers to manage their own care when appropriate.

Platform 6: Improving safety and quality of care

At the point of registration, the registered nurse will be able to:

6.7 understand how the quality and effectiveness of nursing care can be evaluated in practice, and demonstrate how to use service delivery evaluation and audit findings to bring about continuous improvement.

Chapter aims

After reading this chapter, you will be able to:

- define clinical decision-making in evidence-based nursing;
- identify a range of clinical decision-making skills used by nurses;
- relate decision-making skills to different types of evidence;
- apply evidence in planned and unplanned nursing decisions;
- evaluate nursing decisions using the **PERSON evaluation tool**;
- understand professional accountability for nursing decisions.

Introduction

This chapter brings together themes from previous chapters about different types of evidence that inform nursing practice to show how they are applied in everyday decisions and actions. Nurses use clinical decision-making skills all the time, but they may not always be aware of doing so. From judging how to approach a patient who appears upset about something, to taking urgent action to resuscitate a patient who has stopped breathing, effective nursing decisions are life-enhancing and can often be life-saving. Improving nurses' awareness, understanding and expertise in applying clinical decision-making skills is essential in order to provide high-quality, evidence-based nursing. This is reflected in the above Nursing and Midwifery Council's Standards of Proficiency for Registered Nurses (NMC, 2018a), and in a Europe-wide 'Tuning' educational research project that defined a nurse as follows:

> *The nurse is a safe, caring and competent decision maker willing to accept personal and professional accountability for his/her actions and continuous learning. The nurse practises within a statutory framework and code of ethics delivering nursing practice (care) that is appropriately based on research, evidence and critical thinking that effectively responds to the needs of individual clients (patients) and diverse populations.*

(González and Wagenaar, 2003)

The emphasis placed on nurses as competent decision-makers reflects a shift in expectations of nurses from being mainly practically skilled to being both **cognitively** and practically skilled, patient-centred professional carers. This involves being answerable and accountable, being able to explain, justify and defend as necessary the reasons, the supporting evidence and the appropriateness of nursing care decisions and actions. Competent decision-making is an attribute associated with graduate nurses. It also highlights the need for lifelong learning in order for nurses to continually update their knowledge and skills.

This chapter describes and explores what clinical decision-making in evidence-based nursing means, with reference to relevant theory, the author's qualitative research study, and practical examples. In doing so, it relates clinical decision-making to different components of *The influences on and dispositions of an evidence-based nurse* model in Figure 1.1 (p. 24). A 'PERSON' evaluation tool (Standing, 2020) is also presented to evaluate nurses' evidence-based clinical decision-making in caring for patients.

Clinical decision-making skills and associated processes

Clinical decision-making is commonly associated with diagnosing illness and prescribing treatment. However, it is more than that, because unless you switch your brain off when you go to work in a clinical area, everything you do involves making a decision – for example, how you manage your time, interact with patients, relate to other healthcare team members and carry out clinical procedures. To research nurses' decision-making, 20 new nursing students were asked to keep reflective journals about their experience and understanding of acquiring and applying clinical decision-making skills for four years, including their first year as registered nurses (Adult/Mental health/Child). These experiences were explored in a series of four audio-taped semi-structured interviews with each respondent. Ten perceptions of clinical decision-making skills in nursing were identified by analysing recurrent themes in the interview transcripts (see Table 7.1).

Collaborative	Sharing, consulting and agreeing decisions with others, i.e., patients, relatives, nursing colleagues, managers, practice supervisors, other health professionals and other agencies if appropriate, e.g., social worker, home warden, charity worker.
Experience and intuition	Recognising similarities between present and past situations, and being guided by what was effective rather than ineffective before and what feels the right thing to do now, e.g. learning how to attend, listen to, communicate and empathise with others in a relaxed but purposeful way that focuses on their needs.

Confidence	Developing self-assurance from previous achievements, knowledge and skills, plus the strength of supporting evidence that enables explanation, justification and defence of decisions and actions.
Systematic	Using a purposeful, methodical, disciplined problem-solving cycle, including identifying and assessing problems, setting goals and making plans, implementing and evaluating (revising as needed) interventions.
Prioritising	Assessing and managing risks: dealing with urgent before non-urgent patient needs; avoiding causing any further harm to patients.
Observation	Making constant use of senses to look, listen or feel if patients need assistance; monitoring vital signs; recording response to treatment; reviewing results of investigations; reporting any concerns promptly.
Standardised	Applying NHS Trust policies/procedures, evidence-based clinical guidelines and assessment tools, and agreed care plans.
Reflective	Undertaking ongoing individual/collective review of experience to identify insights and address knowledge gaps to inform future care.
Ethical sensitivity	Checking patients are informed and consent to care; communicating 'bad news' sensitively; maintaining duty of care in ethical dilemmas.
Accountability	Ensuring actions are defensible, are in patients' best interests and comply with NMC *Code*, local policy and relevant legislation.

Table 7.1   Perceptions of clinical decision-making skills from student nurse to staff nurse
Source: Standing, 2007, 2010, 2020.

Table 7.1 demonstrates that clinical decision-making in nursing is a multifaceted and complex process. This is because it involves continually combining and applying many different processes in anticipating and responding to the needs of those in your care through timely, well-informed, justifiable actions throughout a period of duty. An extract from one of the above interview transcripts is presented in the following case study, where a student nurse coming to the end of her second Adult Branch placement reflects on an incident in which she felt she had to take the initiative to support the wife of a patient.

Case study: The patient's wife

A gentleman was scheduled for an operation to remove cancer from his bowel and create a colostomy (permanent opening in his abdomen) where a special bag would be attached to collect and dispose of faeces for the rest of his life. He was, naturally, anxious about having such major surgery and his wife came in to comfort him before he went to theatre.

When it was time for him to go, I said to his wife, 'You can go down with him if you like. I'll show you where it is.' I took her along and checked that the receiving theatre staff were happy for her to stay until the anaesthetic was given. When she returned to the ward she sat in a chair by the empty space where her husband's bed had been, looking very worried.

(Continued)

I said, 'Are you OK?' She burst into tears and I knew that she needed someone to spend time with her, so I said, 'Look, I'll go and make a cup of tea.' I pulled the curtains round and we had a cup of tea together (I don't know whether I should have had one, but it felt more natural having a cup of tea together) and a chat. She told me about him and about herself and her family, and after a few tears I put my arm around her. She really was grateful afterwards and said, 'You know, I really needed someone to talk to.' I look back on that and I am so glad I sat and spoke to that woman and that I knew she needed someone to talk to. It could be my mother, you see, and I would hate to think that nobody sat and comforted her. It was basic human rights, common-sense stuff. A year ago, I might not have done that, but I have grown in confidence.

Applying the ten perceptions of clinical decision-making skills to the case study

It is important that nurses can question, examine, explain, justify and defend their decisions and actions when required. The ten perceptions of clinical decision-making skills identified in Table 7.1 offer a useful framework to analyse the nursing student's clinical decision-making skills in the case study, as follows.

Observation: The student nurse noticed how anxious the patient looked prior to surgery, how worried the wife looked on returning to the ward, and how she seemed to benefit from talking to someone.

Experience and intuition: The student nurse knew it was possible for relatives to accompany patients to theatre when she suggested it, and she sensed this was appropriate as the patient was anxious and seemed comforted by the wife's presence. She also understood that the wife had to suppress her own fears about the outcome of surgery and had nobody else to confide in about this.

Collaborative: The student nurse worked in partnership with the patient and his wife to reduce his level of stress prior to surgery. She ensured that the receiving theatre team agreed for the wife to stay until the anaesthetic was given and she made herself available to support the wife if needed.

Ethical sensitivity: The student nurse extended a duty of care to include the wife as well as the patient in recognising her fears about the seriousness and long-term implications of his condition. She was aware it was not accepted practice to stop for a cup of tea and a chat with a relative on a busy ward, but she judged it was appropriate as it was an effective way to offer support.

Prioritising: The student nurse knew that the patient's needs were being addressed in theatre, she had no one else to prepare for surgery and she recognised that the wife might need an opportunity to talk.

Standardised: Preoperative procedures (consent, bath, fasting, medication to relax, check identity tag, vital signs, remove dentures) would have been followed, ensuring the gentleman was ready for surgery.

Systematic: The student nurse demonstrated skilful use of **informative, supportive** and **cathartic interventions** (Heron, 2001) as follows: in letting the wife know she could accompany her husband to theatre (informative); in acknowledging her anxieties, concerns and the need to talk (supportive); and in giving her permission to express her feelings by asking directly 'Are you OK?' and then reassuring her that she had time to listen (cathartic).

Accountability: The supervising staff nurse is technically accountable for care given by the student, but their main priority was pre- and post-operative patient care. The student's sense of responsibility for supporting the patient's wife is endorsed by the NMC professional *Code*, which states that you should *recognise when people are anxious or in distress and respond compassionately and politely* (NMC, 2018b, p7).

Reflective: The student nurse applied **reflection-in-action** in taking the initiative to facilitate the wife to accompany the patient to theatre and in responding to her apparent distress when she returned. Looking back, she used **reflection-on-action** in affirming the importance of supporting relatives.

Confidence: The student nurse had grown in confidence in her decision-making and interpersonal skills in recognising and addressing the wife's unmet needs, and achieving a successful outcome.

Having applied the ten perceptions of clinical decision-making to review the nursing student's interventions in the case study, it begs the question – so what? Is it a case of over-theorising and over-analysing a relatively straightforward and common-sense example of good nursing practice? Or does the application of such frameworks (informed by and developed from research evidence) tell us something important about the nature of clinical decision-making in evidence-based nursing practice?

Activity 7.1   Critical thinking

One way for you to assess the usefulness of the ten perceptions of clinical decision-making is to consider whether or not they promote the development and application of the essential 'dispositions of the evidence-based nurse' identified in Chapter 1 (Figure 1.1). These are listed below. Look again at the ten perceptions of clinical decision-making and try to match them to any of the dispositions you think they relate to, with reference to appropriate examples from the case study where possible.

(Continued)

Dispositions of the evidence-based nurse	Perceptions of clinical decision-making relating to the dispositions	Examples in the case study of linking the dispositions and perceptions
• Other regarding		
• Engaged with self		
• Questioning		
• Reflective		
• Reflexive		
• Creative thinker		
• Critical thinker		
• Morally active		

Some possible outline answers are provided at the end of the chapter.

So far, this chapter has described different aspects (perceptions) of clinical decision-making and suggested that they relate to different qualities (dispositions) of nurses in evidence-based practice. Later on in the chapter, the ten perceptions of clinical decision-making will be related to the different types of evidence identified in Chapter 1. Before moving on to that, it is worth spending a bit more time thinking about other characteristics of clinical decision-making highlighted in the case study. The case study illustrates a contrast between nursing decisions and actions that are planned and those that are unplanned. Preoperative nursing care of the patient would have been a well-planned and standardised procedure, whereas noticing and responding to the patient's and his wife's fear and anxiety was a spontaneous or unplanned reaction that applied experience and intuition. The relatively high level of contact that nurses have with patients, relatives, friends and carers (compared to many other professions) means that they get more opportunities for both planned and unplanned clinical decision-making. Are you aware of how much time you spend on planned as opposed to unplanned nursing care?

Activity 7.2 Reflection

Identify a day in your clinical placement to do a time-and-motion study of everything you do, from the moment you arrive to the moment you leave the clinical area. Take a notebook with you to record events and their duration during your shift, if possible (so you don't have to try to recall everything at the end of the day). Review the day's activities and calculate how much time was spent on planned (e.g., agreed care plan) versus unplanned (e.g., responding to situations that arise) decisions and associated patient care. Match each example to the ten perceptions of clinical decision-making skills as appropriate for both planned and unplanned care. Reflect on whether the ten perceptions apply equally to planned and unplanned decisions and related nursing care.

Some possible answers can be found at the end of the chapter.

Sometimes nursing interventions need to combine elements of both planned and unplanned decision-making. For example, our duty to ensure patient safety means that potential unexpected events such as a fire, an accident in a clinical area, a medical emergency or dealing with an aggressive incident must be anticipated. Contingency plans such as a fire drill must be made, ready to put into effect when required. It is important that you discuss with your practice supervisor what is expected of you and your role in such circumstances. Ask to see policies and procedures for managing such events so you are familiar with them and take part in any drills and training events to practise procedures and help to develop the necessary skills.

Activity 7.3   Research and finding out

Look through the various emergency guidelines and procedures in your clinical placement and see if you can identify examples of the ten perceptions of clinical decision-making skills being applied.

Identify any of the ten perceptions of clinical decision-making skills that you feel should be applied in all situations (including carefully planned care, spontaneous unplanned care and implementing procedures for emergencies) and write down why you think they are important. Check whether your fellow students, qualified nurse colleagues or practice supervisor agree or disagree with your choices.

Some possible answers can be found at the end of the chapter.

Defining clinical decision-making in nursing

Decision-making involves choosing what action to take from the available alternatives and then carrying it out. In its most basic form, it means choosing to do something or choosing not to do it – for example, washing your hands before cooking a meal or not (in which case not washing your hands is an alternative action, albeit passive) and saying 'yes' or 'no' when someone offers you a cup of tea. Decision-making, therefore, employs thinking skills to exercise judgement in assessing the benefits of possible options and choosing a preferred option that is then acted upon. Clinical decision-making refers to decisions made by health professionals in the course of their work in promoting health, diagnosing or treating disease, relieving suffering and caring for patients. Becoming skilled in clinical decision-making requires the application of a range of evidence regarding patient concerns, physical and human resources within healthcare contexts, understanding health and illness, developing expertise in applying therapeutic approaches, a commitment to enhance the well-being of those in your care and fulfilling the requirements of the relevant professional body.

Clinical decision-making in nursing refers to any decisions made by nurses in choosing how to deliver care to patients for whom they are responsible. The Nursing and Midwifery Council is the professional body that specifies education requirements for entry to the register as a qualified nurse and for maintaining registration status. It also regulates the profession through publishing a code of conduct that nurses must comply with or face potential disciplinary action. For example: *We can take action if registered nurses or midwives fail to uphold the Code. In serious cases, this can include removing them from the register* (NMC, 2018b, p3). Making the wrong clinical decisions is, therefore, not only potentially harmful to patients, but it may also call into question your continuing practice as a nurse. Learning about, developing and applying effective clinical decision-making skills is vital for the well-being of patients and nurses' capacity to demonstrate that decisions are justified. The following definition summarises key elements of clinical decision-making in nursing.

> *Clinical decision-making is a complex process involving observation, information processing, critical thinking, evaluating evidence, applying relevant knowledge, problem solving skills, reflection and clinical judgement to select the best course of action which optimises a patient's health and minimises any potential harm. The role of the clinical decision-maker in nursing is, therefore, to be professionally accountable for accurately assessing patients' needs using appropriate sources of information, and planning nursing interventions that address problems and which they are competent to perform.*

(Standing, 2007, 2010)

This definition emphasises that clinical decisions:

- are patient-centred in anticipating and responding to patients'/service users' needs to address their health problems;
- involve identifying, reviewing and applying relevant information from different sources – for example, observations, the patient's story, clinical guidelines, theory and research evidence;
- require the application of cognitive skills such as problem solving, critical thinking, reflection and judgement in selecting the best option;
- are associated with delivering competent, effective nursing care for which nurses are accountable.

In this way, clinical decision-making reflects the notion of evidence-based nursing, as described and advocated throughout this book. These skills are central to nurses' professional identity, as stated in the definition of a nurse (González and Wagenaar, 2003) presented at the beginning of this chapter. In Activity 7.4 you are asked to apply aspects of the above definition to reflect on your own experience of clinical decision-making.

Activity 7.4 Reflection

Next time you are in a clinical practice setting, make a point of noting down all the decisions that relate to patient care that *you* have to make during your shift. Later, when you have time, reflect on these decisions, then try to answer the following questions.

1. In what way were your decisions relevant to the needs of the patients you cared for?
2. What type of evidence did you refer to and how did this influence your decision-making?
3. What types of thinking skills did you apply?
4. How did you evaluate the outcomes of your decisions?

As this is based on your own reflections, there is no outline answer at the end of the chapter.

Applying different types of evidence in nursing decisions

Evidence refers to information that is used to support particular beliefs, decisions and actions. It can be sensory – for example, feeling tired and hungry at the end of 'a long day' at work and deciding to stop at a favourite eating place on the way home rather than cook something yourself. It can be emotional – for example, feeling sad or angry about something that happened and deciding to talk to a sympathetic friend to 'get it off your chest'. It can be practical – for example, you notice that your front door has begun to squeak annoyingly when opened or closed, so you decide to oil its hinges. It can be theoretical – for example, planning a holiday abroad and deciding to read up on the history, customs and culture, and places of interest to visit. It can be technological – for example, needing to ensure that information on the home computer is not lost if the system 'crashes' and deciding to install a back-up external hard drive. It can also be scientific – for example, understanding that water conducts electricity and deciding to dry your hands and body before switching on the hairdryer to reduce the risk of an electric shock. In the above examples personal decisions, subsequent actions and their potential consequences are prompted by knowledge and understanding derived from a wide range of information sources or types of evidence. The same is true of nursing decisions.

Earlier chapters looked in detail at different types of evidence in nursing. Chapter 1 summarised these in Figure 1.1 (p24). In order to see how different types of evidence may influence nursing decisions, Table 7.2 suggests possible matches with the ten perceptions of clinical decision-making skills described earlier.

Applying research evidence to systematic and standardised decision-making

Research evidence is often seen as the essential basis of high-quality, evidence-based healthcare because it involves rigorous testing of the validity and reliability of methods used and reported findings, which are open to critical scrutiny and testing by

Evidence influencing practice	Associated clinical decision-making skills
Research evidence	Systematic, standardised
Practice knowledge	Observation, reflective
Experience	Experience and intuition, confidence
Policy	Prioritising, standardised
Resources	Prioritising, accountability
Patient preference	Collaborative, ethical sensitivity
Views of other professionals	Collaborative, experience and intuition
Ethics	Ethical sensitivity, accountability
Law	Accountability, standardised

Table 7.2 Different types of evidence informing clinical decision-making skills in nursing

others (see Chapters 3 and 4). This scientific (physical and social) approach to generating new knowledge has influenced the development of systematic problem solving and associated decision-making – for example, the nursing process (ongoing cycle of assessment, planning, implementation and evaluation of care – 'APIE'). In many clinical areas, the use of the nursing process is standardised, meaning it is adopted as a framework for all nurses to use in delivering and recording care. Some use 'ASPIRE', which adds two stages – 'systematic nursing diagnosis' and 'recheck' – to the nursing process. To guide nurses in targeting systematic care, the nursing process is often used in conjunction with the Activities of Living model (Roper et al., 2000; Holland et al., 2019; Wilson et al., 2018) to assess patients' abilities and needs in 12 areas (maintaining a safe environment; communicating; breathing; eating and drinking; eliminating; personal cleansing and dressing; controlling body temperature; mobilising; working and playing; expressing sexuality; sleeping; preparing for dying). In effect, this is a checklist of patients' general physical, psychological and social health and well-being to help nurses provide comprehensive person-centred assessment and care to address health concerns in partnership with patients.

Research evidence also informs clinical guidelines produced by the National Institute for Health and Care Excellence (NICE) in caring for particular patients with specific needs and health problems – for example, those suffering from COVID-19 infection (NICE, 2021). There will be NICE clinical guidelines relating to whichever area of practice you are working. NICE clinical guidelines are being continually developed, applied to patient care and updated.

Case study: Care of patients who have learning disabilities and suffer from epilepsy

The NICE Guideline – NG217 – Epilepsies in children, young people and adults (NICE, 2022) assists nurses and other health professionals in caring for those suffering from various forms of epilepsy (neurological abnormality associated with involuntary seizures (fits) and/ or loss of consciousness). People with learning disabilities are on average 20 times more likely to suffer from epilepsy than the general population. A study was therefore set up to compare care for this group of vulnerable patients, before and after a previous edition (CG20) of these guidelines were implemented. The results of the study are summarised below.

Implementing NICE guideline CG20 for the management of epilepsy in a learning disability service.

	Before implementation %	After implementation %
Proportion of patients whose seizures were accurately described and classified	6	83
Proportion where frequency of seizures was recorded	81	100
Proportion where severity of seizures was recorded	57	100
Proportion of changes made to seizure diagnosis	0	76
Proportion of individualised risk assessment carried out	4.5	100
Medical consultations led to changes in treatment plans	50	91

The above case study illustrates how evidence-based, standardised clinical guidelines can help healthcare practitioners to work more systematically in identifying and managing health problems. It indicated that assessment of patients' symptoms became much more accurate and comprehensive, which in turn informed changes to patients' diagnosis, risk management and medical treatment. Such guidelines not only inform medical treatment, but they also influence nurses' decision-making and offer information for service users and/or their families to understand the options available to them. It also shows that clinical guidelines are always evolving following a review of their application in order to update evidence-based care.

Activity 7.5   Decision-making

Although epilepsy may be more common in people with learning disabilities, it can affect anyone, including people with mental health problems, children and adults throughout the population. Whichever pathway you are practising in, it is therefore important that you know how to assess and manage various health risks associated with this condition. Use the 12 areas (listed above) in the Activities of Living model (Roper et al., 2000; Holland

(Continued)

and Jenkins, 2019; Wilson et al., 2018) as a checklist for a risk assessment of someone having a generalised tonic-clonic seizure with impaired consciousness and say how you would manage the risks during and following tonic (involuntary muscle rigidity) and clonic (involuntary alternating muscle contractions) phases of the seizure.

Some possible answers can be found at the end of the chapter.

Applying practice knowledge to observation and reflective decision-making

While research evidence is usually documented, made explicit and widely disseminated, practice knowledge refers to localised, context-specific skills and tacit understanding – for example, the **embedded knowledge** within customs and practices that distinguish one clinical placement from another. Practice knowledge includes technical skills such as the dexterity to do an aseptic wound dressing, interpersonal skills in being attentive and listening to patients' concerns, and noticing changes in behaviour that signal someone needs attention (as the student did in the patient's wife case study). In the following case study, a surgical nurse intervenes when a patient complains of pain in a limb he no longer has.

Case study: Phantom pain

Following surgery, a gentleman who smoked heavily for 40 years and who suffers from peripheral vascular disease (poor circulation affecting feet and legs) and diabetes, is distressed by pains he feels come from his right foot following below-knee amputation of his right leg, which had been gangrenous. Through reflection-in-action, the surgical nurse understands that this is phantom limb pain (PLP) which 50–85 per cent of patients experience as real, sometimes severe pain following amputation, which they may find disturbing (Colquhoun et al., 2019). The gentleman is offered painkillers as prescribed and is reassured that what he is experiencing is not unusual, that the pains should gradually subside and that the science behind this phenomenon is not yet fully understood. The surgical nurse also checks with the anaesthetist whether alternative post-operative pain relief is needed, such as an anaesthetic nerve block that is administered continuously via a catheter (Neil, 2016).

Reflecting back on such encounters with patients (reflection-on-action) enables nurses to link clinical experience to relevant theory or research evidence. We can do this by finding answers to questions arising from our observations and practical understanding of patients' needs. In the above case study, the surgical nurse understood that phantom pain can be severe and questioned if the patient's prescribed pain management is sufficient. An alternative research question could be, 'Might visualisation and virtual massage of amputated limbs help to relieve phantom pains experienced by amputees?' Where appropriate research-based treatments and procedures are discovered and implemented, their effectiveness needs to be evaluated by applying practice knowledge using observation and communication skills to reflect on care outcomes with patients. Hence, reflection-on-action may also help to articulate hidden valuable practice knowledge or skills embedded in clinical areas and make it explicit, thereby contributing to the development of nursing theory.

Activity 7.6   Reflection

Identify a clinical placement that you have been allocated to and try to identify specific practice knowledge you associate with experienced nurses in that particular area of patient care.

- What technical and practical knowledge and skills do the nurses apply?
- What interpersonal and communication skills do you notice the nurses using?
- What observation skills do nurses demonstrate in that clinical area?
- What examples of the nurses' reflective clinical decision-making have you witnessed?
- Talk to your practice supervisor about how you can develop your practice knowledge and related skills.

As this activity is based on your own reflection, there is no outline answer at the end of the chapter.

Applying experience to experience and intuition and confidence in decision-making

Experience refers to an accumulation of personal embodied knowledge that incorporates an individual's unique interpretation of their role as a nurse; interpersonal relationships with patients, staff and others; theoretical and research input; and influential life events. Connecting these disparate influences defines a nurse's personal and professional identity, which the individual draws upon in subconsciously recognising patterns in information cues to facilitate their intuitive judgement. In a sense, this is what happens between people who have intimate mutual understanding and, without prompting, know what the other person is thinking or feeling. Developing and confidently using this skill as a nurse in quickly assessing a crisis situation, understanding what needs to done and organising an effective, speedy resolution is associated with expert practitioners (Benner, 1984). This is the most difficult type of decision to explain because it may be based on a hunch or feeling that is only justified where there is a positive outcome. However, this type of decision is prone to error – for example, you might believe a parent who says her child tripped while playing, only to discover later that it was a non-accidental injury from physical abuse. It is, therefore, advisable to test out intuitions – for example, by seeking out a second opinion from an experienced colleague.

Activity 7.7   Communication

Test out your intuitive abilities with a group of colleagues at college or in the clinical area.

- Each person privately thinks of a living creature they feel they can strongly identify with.
- Everyone writes (in BLOCK CAPITALS to reduce handwriting recognition) the name of their chosen creature on the same type/size paper and all the names are put into a hat.
- Someone makes a list of all the creatures identified in the hat for everyone to share (if two people happen to identify the same creature, then list it twice).
- Each person then privately writes down which group member they feel most closely characterises each living creature.
- Everyone goes through the list of creatures together to see how many guesses were right and how many were wrong.

As this activity is based on your own engagement with the activity, there is no outline answer at the end of the chapter.

Applying policy to prioritising and standardised decision-making

Following the Health and Social Care Act 2012 and 2022, health policy priorities and NHS funding have been set by the Department of Health and Social Care in England and by the respective government departments of Scotland, Wales and Northern Ireland. Adding Social Care to the Department of Health's responsibilities recognises that caring for people's health and welfare is not solely confined to the NHS as individual members of the public, community groups, charities, social services and local government all make a contribution. A policy emerged of creating Integrated Care Systems where the various agencies work together to be more efficient and responsive to local communities' needs in promoting health, preventing illness and addressing both acute and long-term care needs more effectively. The NHS Long Term Plan (NHS, 2019) applied policy priorities by shifting the emphasis from traditional hospital-orientated treatment to a preventative, community-orientated, person-centred, accessible, evidence-based, innovative and integrated system of healthcare.

Reducing health inequalities by helping everyone to live longer, healthier lives with clean air and water, good nutrition, exercise and less smoking, alcohol or drug dependence is a recurring aim of health policy. Reducing morbidity and mortality from circulatory disease, cancer or diabetes by screening of those at risk and early intervention as necessary also remains a priority. This is complemented by digital technology, including the NHS App, for the public to engage directly in monitoring their own healthcare. They can also raise concerns about quality of health and social care via local 'Healthwatch' watchdogs. Translating health policy into prioritising and standardised decision-making is enabled by the National Institute for Health Research (NIHR) projects, like the development of the AstraZeneca COVID-19 vaccine that was a product of such research and, together with other vaccines, helped to significantly reduce rates and severity of COVID infections. Hence, NIHR produces valuable research that may be incorporated within evidence-based NICE clinical guidelines to improve quality of care – for example, care of patients debilitated by COVID-19 (NICE, 2021).

Applying resources to prioritising and accountability in decision-making

Making decisions about people's care is dependent on having the necessary resources in terms of the funds, organisational structure, materials and workforce to do so. The main source of funding for healthcare is income tax and national insurance contributions. The Treasury allocates the Department of Health and Social Care an annual budget, most of which is given to UK national NHS bodies who in turn allocate most of it to Integrated Care Systems (ICSs) according to the size, demography and health needs of the local populations they serve. Integrated Care Boards (ICBs) purchase services from providers such as hospitals, GPs or health centres to address the identified healthcare needs within their allocated budget (King's Fund, 2022).

Hence, the financial resources needed to sustain a 'cradle-to-grave' national system of healthcare, that is free at the point of delivery, depends on having a strong economy. Making the best use of the funds available depends on the efficient organisation of services in providing the facilities needed and skilled workforce required to address health priorities. If the organisational structure is overly bureaucratic, then policy and decision-making is 'top down', so less in tune with patients' needs and the challenges that practitioners face. It also means that administrative costs are 'top heavy', thereby diverting funds from patient care. The Health and Social Care Act 2012/2022 and Long Term NHS Plan 2019 looked at reducing bureaucracy by involving clinicians in the commissioning of care responsive to local needs. Just as health professionals are accountable to professional bodies, NHS Trusts and social care providers are assessed by the Care Quality Commission (CQC) as satisfactory or unsatisfactory in delivering compassionate, high-quality evidence-based care. If they do not make improvements specified by the CQC, they can lose contracts and be prevented from carrying on.

The global Coronavirus pandemic placed considerable strain on the NHS's ability to cope with high infection rates and those requiring acute critical care. Resources were diverted away from previous priority areas, resulting in many services being curtailed and the build-up of an extensive backlog of patients awaiting treatment for other conditions. The success of the COVID-19 vaccination programme gives an opportunity to reflect on any lessons to be learned. The King's Fund (2021) urges governments to focus on five priorities.

1.   Putting the workforce centre stage.
2.   A step change on inequalities and population health.
3.   Lasting reform for social care.
4.   Embedding and accelerating digital change.
5.   Reshaping the relationship between communities and public services.

Hence, COVID-19 has highlighted: 1) the value of the NHS workforce; 2) inequalities in the health of ethnic minorities and vulnerable elderly within social care; and 3) success in bringing communities and services together and the use of technology in socially distanced consultations.

Applying patient preference to collaborative and ethical sensitivity in decision-making

The Department of Health and Social Care and NHS Trusts advocate high-quality patient-centred care, greater treatment choice, invite verbal, written or online feedback from patients about their experiences, and have policies in place that are intended to deal with patients' or relatives' complaints promptly and thoroughly. It is, therefore, important for nurses not simply to listen to patients' preferences or queries regarding their care, but to respond appropriately in respecting their views and addressing their concerns.

In some situations, patient preference is not catered for because of financial constraints and geographical variations in policy. For example, new drugs prolonging the lives of those suffering from cancer are not available in some NHS Trusts because they are considered too expensive, but in others the same drugs are freely available. Sometimes patients do not want the NHS to prolong their lives and refuse treatment, presenting healthcare professionals with an ethical dilemma.

Case study: Refusal of treatment

A frail 98-year-old patient, who has outlived all her relatives and friends, stopped eating a week ago and says she does not want to be fed by any alternative means. If the healthcare team do not intervene, they will be respecting her wishes but contributing to her starvation and potential premature death. If they decide to feed her with supplements via intravenous infusion, they will be going against her wishes but will probably extend her sad and lonely life.

Activity 7.8   Reflection

If you were a member of the healthcare team in the case study above – Refusal of treatment – which one of the options would you support? What is the rationale to justify your choice of action?

The actual answer reached by the team is referred to in the next section for your information.

Sometimes patients take more direct action to end their lives. For example, a young man being treated for depression in an acute mental health unit says goodnight to the new night nurse and goes to bed. When the nurse goes round checking on patients an hour later, he discovers the young man dead underneath the covers having tied a plastic bag over his head. The nurse feels terribly guilty for not taking more time to talk to the patient and for not checking on him sooner. These feelings are exacerbated as the police and coroner investigate the death (ruling out homicide), by the parents' grief at losing their son when they thought he was being safely looked after, and in having to describe and explain his actions to hospital managers.

Activity 7.9   Reflection

Do you agree with the nurse that he could have prevented the young man's suicide if he had been more vigilant? Do you think the nurse was particularly negligent in the standard of care offered? What evidence might have been helpful in alerting the nurse to observe the young man closely?

There are some possible answers and thoughts at the end of the chapter.

Applying views, experience and intuition to collaborative decision-making

The dilemma presented by the elderly lady refusing food requires careful consideration and collaboration between the patient, nurses, doctors and managers. One nurse had formed a good relationship with the patient through spending time with her, listening and talking to her about her past, how she is feeling now, her likes and dislikes, and her refusal to accept nutrients. Sometimes the lady agreed to sip a cup of tea or, with encouragement, to nibble on a biscuit, but it was not enough to sustain her. In contributing to a team discussion, the nurse said she did not agree with intravenous feeding because it would upset the lady and deny her the dignity of choosing how to spend the remainder of her life. Others felt uncomfortable that this could be seen as neglect and that every effort should be made to keep her alive. Some wondered whether the lady might not be mentally competent to make a decision and thought the team ought to make one for her in the absence of relatives. However, the nurse argued that the lady was quite lucid, not confused, sad but not severely depressed, and it would be uncaring to force her into actions that would prolong her life against her wishes. The team finally agreed that they would respect the patient's wishes by not feeding her artificially (intravenously) but that the nurses would continue offering her food and drink, and someone to talk to. Pooling experiences and views to debate patient care in this way is a valuable way of promoting effective teamwork. Teamwork enables learning from different perspectives and disciplines, feeling valued and recognised by interprofessional colleagues, and co-ordinating and integrating an effective system of care delivery tailored to the individual patient's unique needs.

Activity 7.10   Research and finding out

Research the Tony Bland case (the case of a young man left in a coma from crush injuries from the Hillsborough Football Stadium disaster in 1989), which set a legal precedent classifying artificial nutrition as medical treatment that doctors (in collaboration with others) could decide whether to give or not. The House of Commons Medical Treatment (Prevention of Euthanasia) Bill (2000) is a useful information source.

As this activity involves your own research, there is no outline answer at the end of the chapter.

Applying ethics to ethical sensitivity and accountability in decision-making

As described in Figure 1.1 (p24), ethical principles (respect for human rights, commitment to good practice, avoidance of harm and treatment of all patients fairly) underpin high-quality, patient-centred, evidence-based nursing. As referred to earlier, the NMC is the professional body that sets out the ethical code of conduct that nurses in the UK must comply with. Good practice – for example, the student nurse being sensitive to the wife of a cancer patient in the first case study in this chapter – exemplifies the application of ethical principles, while poor practice – for example, patients being left in badly soiled bed-linen – is in breach of all the above principles, and *The Code* (NMC, 2018b). In order to maintain public trust and the right to remain on the nursing register, nurses must always conduct themselves in a caring, professional, well-informed and competent manner. Where this is found not to be the case, nurses are held to account for their behaviour and disciplined, which can include being removed from the NMC register and forfeiting the right to work as a registered nurse.

Case studies: Examples of misconduct

These are examples of nurses who received 'Striking Off Orders' from the NMC register at the Conduct and Competence Committee hearings (September 2015) when their fitness to practise was found to be currently impaired.

- An adult medical unit nurse failed to carry out appropriate safety checks prior to the administration of blood, resulting in the wrong blood transfusion being given to a patient. The nurse also failed to undertake and/or document appropriate observations of the patient after administering the wrong blood transfusion.
- A learning disabilities community nurse failed to visit certain patients in the community when it was her duty to do so. The nurse failed to record visits or write appropriate care plans for patients who had been seen. The nurse also failed to ensure that risk assessment documents were completed and failed to request further diagnostic tests and a 'CT' head scan needed to assess risks to patients' health.
- A mental health nurse was convicted under the Sexual Offences Act 2003 and imprisoned for: 1) Causing or inciting a child to engage in sexual activity, contrary to section 10(1); 2) Meeting a child following sexual grooming, contrary to section 15(1); 3) Sexual activity with a child, contrary to section 9 (1). The nurse met the victim at an amateur dramatic group and the crimes occurred outside of work, but the serious nature of the offences meant that the nurse was found unsuitable to remain on the register.
- A children's nurse prepared a child for surgery, including administering premedication despite knowing that the child had recently eaten, which made it unsafe to operate at that time. The nurse failed to carry out appropriate post-operative observations. The nurse also failed to escalate concerns to medical staff when a child's Paediatric Advanced Warning Score (PAWS) of 4 indicated that this was necessary.

Applying law to accountability and standardised decision-making

The NMC is empowered under the terms of Nursing and Midwifery Order 2001 legislation to safeguard the health and well-being of the public and regulate the profession. Similarly, nursing students have to demonstrate good health, good character and fitness to practise, and to declare any police cautions, charges or criminal convictions to ensure that patients are protected (NMC, 2019).

The law, specifically the Health and Safety at Work Act 1974, can protect all nurses in the workplace by requiring employers to take measures (training, equipment, procedures) to control risks to their health and safety. Employees also have a responsibility to report safety concerns; arguably, the nurses at the NHS Trust referred to earlier had sufficient grounds to report serious health risks regarding infection-control systems, procedures and associated staffing problems.

The law can also be used to protect all patients. For example, the Data Protection Act 2018 (OPSI, 2018) requires confidential patient information to be kept securely and accessed only by authorised personnel. Nurses need to think about the implications of this legislation in their everyday practice – for example, when asking patients about their personal details, given that the rise in identity fraud highlights risks associated with a lack of privacy.

Scenario

A patient attends an outpatient clinic for an appointment with a consultant to review recent tests of her heart and lung function. The waiting room is full of other patients, but the experienced nurse loudly and unceremoniously asks her to confirm her full name, address, date of birth, telephone number, work contact details and next of kin, then weighs her and announces the result for all to hear.

In the above scenario, the patient's confidential information was not kept securely and was accessible to non-authorised personnel, contrary to the Data Protection Act 1998. It is also a breach of section 5.1 of *The Code, respect a person's right to privacy in all aspects of their care* (NMC, 2018b, p8). The experienced nurse should have therefore ensured that the interview was conducted discreetly and sensitively.

Under the terms of the Freedom of Information Act 2000, the public have the right to see any records made by nurses or others regarding their care. Hence, it is important for nurses to remember that relevant sections of case notes and reflective portfolios they have compiled could be accessed and scrutinised by patients and their legal representatives.

Some laws relate to specific groups of service users. For example, the Children Act 1989 (OPSI, 1989) specifies that if you have reason to suspect that a child has been physically, emotionally or sexually abused, you must report it straightaway to social services who are obliged to investigate and, if necessary, remove the child to a place of safety. With mentally ill patients, there may be a double risk regarding self-harm or sometimes a possibility of harming others. The Mental Health Act 1983 specifies criteria for the voluntary or compulsory treatment of patients according to the perceived type, level and duration of risk to themselves or others, to protect both patients and the public. The Mental Capacity Act 2005 protects people who are unable to make decisions, and requires nurses and others who have a duty of care to act in their best interests.

Evaluating evidence-based nursing decisions using 'PERSON'

We have seen that the ten perceptions of clinical decision-making identified by nurses (Standing, 2007, 2010, 2020) can be related to the nine different forms of evidence described in this book. This may be helpful to you if you are asked to explain the rationale and evidence-base of your own nursing decisions. Registered nurses are obliged to ask themselves this question every time they make a clinical decision because they are professionally accountable for delivering safe and effective person-centred, evidence-based patient care. The 'PERSON' evaluation tool described in Table 7.3 has been developed to help nurses and midwives evaluate their clinical decisions.

Whichever perceptions of clinical decision-making that you are applying (e.g., 'collaborative', 'ethical sensitivity') you can evaluate your decisions using the 'PERSON' evaluation tool. Similarly, 'PERSON' offers a structure to harness the dispositions of the evidence-based nurse (Chapter 1) to evaluate your clinical decision-making. For example, the 'other regarding' and 'morally active' dispositions correspond to the 'Patient-centred' element of 'PERSON'. By answering the questions in the right-hand column, you are prompted to critically reflect on your decisions and associated care regarding each element of the evaluation tool. In doing so, you will be generating evidence of your commitment to achieve high-quality, patient-centred, evidence-based care. This is important because it can help you to demonstrate your accountability for meeting the professional standards in *The Code* (NMC, 2018b) which requires you to 1) prioritise people; 2) practise effectively; 3) preserve safety; and 4) promote professionalism and trust.

'PERSON' acronym	Answer these questions to evaluate your decisions
Patient-centred	Were different care options explained to the patient?
(Prioritise people)	Did the patient give consent before the intervention?
	How did the patient's opinion contribute to care plans?
	If for any reason the patient was unable to contribute to decisions, how were his or her rights safeguarded?
Evidence-based	What patient observations indicated a need for action?
(Practise effectively)	What corroborating evidence supports your assessment?
	What was the rationale for the selected intervention?
	What research evidence underpins the intervention?
Risks assessed and managed	What threats to patient's health/well-being were there?
	What was done to ensure a safe healthcare environment?
	What procedure did you follow to control known risks?
	How did you escalate concerns if problems worsened?

(Continued)

Table 7.3 (Continued)

'PERSON' acronym	Answer these questions to evaluate your decisions
Safe and effective delivery of care *(Preserve safety)*	What knowledge/skills/attitudes were applied to care?
	What prior experience did you have of this intervention?
	How was your competence to give care quality assured?
	How did you share information on the care you gave?
Outcomes of care benefit the patient	What was the patient's/relatives' feedback about care?
	To what extent were desired outcomes of care achieved?
	How do you think the patient benefitted from this care?
	How will you address any negative outcomes of care?
Nursing and midwifery strengths and weaknesses *(Promote professionalism and trust)*	What did you learn from this experience of patient care?
	How did you justify public trust in your ability to care?
	On reflection, what could you have done differently?
	What are you doing to improve your decision-making skills?

Table 7.3 Clinical decision-making 'PERSON' evaluation tool

Standing, 2020, pp246–7.

In Table 7.4, 'PERSON' is applied to evaluate the nurse's contribution to the team's decision-making regarding the case study, Refusal of treatment, discussed earlier in the chapter (p140).

PATIENT-CENTRED
Were different care options explained to the patient? When the 98-year-old lady stopped eating and drinking, she was offered an intravenous infusion of fluids/nutritional supplements, and the consequences of dehydration and starvation were explained.
Did the patient give consent before the intervention? The lady refused to accept being fed artificially via an infusion.
How did the patient's opinion contribute to care plans? The patient's preference for not being fed via an infusion was discussed by the healthcare team. The nurse advocated on behalf of the patient that she should not be force-fed against her will. The team agreed not to administer nutrients via infusion, but to offer fluids/food by mouth and someone for the patient to talk to.
If for any reason the patient was unable to contribute to decisions, how were his or her rights safeguarded? The healthcare team questioned whether the lady had the mental capacity to fully understand the risks to her health and well-being, from her lack of adequate nourishment. If it was thought that she was confused or depressed, then it could be argued that the team were obligated to take action to safeguard her health/well-being by feeding her without her consent (she had no living relatives to involve in decision-making). The nurse who had been looking after the lady argued that she was very lucid and on this basis her preferences should be respected.
EVIDENCE-BASED
What patient observations indicated a need for action? The lady had stopped eating or drinking sufficient amounts to nourish herself adequately. She was losing weight and becoming progressively weaker.

What corroborating evidence supports your assessment? When presented with food and drink, the lady would ignore it. If the nurse spent time talking to her, she could persuade her to sip fluids or nibble on a biscuit but no more than that.

What was the rationale for the selected intervention? To respect the patient's wish to refuse food/fluids via infusion (despite knowing this could hasten her death) in order for her to be allowed a dignified way of ending 98 years of life on her own terms.

What research evidence underpins the intervention? A survey of hospice nurses in the USA reported that the vast majority of end-of-life care patients who chose to stop food and fluids because they felt ready for their lives to end, died peacefully and with dignity within 15 days of doing so (Ganzini et al., 2003).

RISKS ASSESSED AND MANAGED

What threats to patient's health/well-being were there? By voluntarily refusing food and drink, the patient's life was at risk, but the alternative of artificially hydrating/feeding her would be against her wishes and threatened her sense of well-being.

What was done to ensure a safe healthcare environment? Ensuring that the lady fully understood the implications and likely consequences of her preferred treatment option, and the potential benefits of alternative options that were available to her.

What procedure did you follow to control known risks? The nurse had established a good rapport with the lady and this enabled her to assess how she was feeling and whether she felt like accepting oral fluids and food offered on a regular basis.

How did you escalate concerns if problems worsened? The nurse's main concern was to fulfil the wishes of the 98-year-old lady. When the healthcare team were considering feeding the lady against her will, the nurse advocated strongly on her behalf.

SAFE AND EFFECTIVE DELIVERY OF CARE

What knowledge/skills/attitudes were applied to care? Principles of patient-centred care, valuing and incorporating patient preference in care planning. Understanding physical (nutrition), psychological (self-determination) and social (companionship) needs. Applying such knowledge in clinical practice by demonstrating ethical sensitivity and collaborative clinical decision-making skills.

What prior experience did you have of this intervention? Third-year student nurse on an Adult pathway who had not encountered an ethical dilemma like this before, but did have previous healthcare assistant experience in mental health.

How was your competence to give care quality assured? The student was mentored and supervised by registered nurses and her clinical competence in caring for patients was formally scrutinised and evaluated in summative practice assessments.

How did you share information on the care you gave? The student told the healthcare team what she had learned from the patient and recorded her interventions in the care plan. She also kept a reflective journal of her understanding of acquiring and applying clinical decision-making skills in nursing in her role as a respondent in a longitudinal qualitative research study (Standing, 2007, 2010, 2020).

OUTCOMES OF CARE BENEFIT THE PATIENT

What was the patient's/relatives' feedback about care? The patient was content that her wishes were respected.

To what extent were desired outcomes of care achieved? The patient was not subjected to invasive techniques to extend her life against her will, which would have prolonged her suffering, and she was supported in achieving a dignified end to her life.

(Continued)

Table 7.4 (Continued)

How do you think the patient benefitted from this care? The lady had no one to care for her, she had formed an attachment with the nurse, she knew she had not long to live, and she felt comfortable ending her life in the care of the healthcare team.
How will you address any negative outcomes of care? It is important to document everything carefully to show that the care delivered was justified and in the patient's best interests. In the UK, it is illegal to assist a person to commit suicide and there is a 'fine line' between not intervening to prolong end-of-life care when patients choose to stop eating and drinking as part of the dying process (Stängle et al., 2019) and what might be perceived as neglect. Hence, the importance of continuing to offer fluids, food and nursing care to the lady so that she could decide whether or not to accept them.
NURSING AND MIDWIFERY STRENGTHS AND WEAKNESSES
What did you learn from this experience of patient care? The student nurse learnt that quality of life was more important to the lady than how much longer she might live, and she learned to be an advocate in conveying the lady's wishes to the team.
How did you justify public trust in your ability to care? The student's decisions and actions preceded publication of the '6Cs' of compassionate care and yet were consistent with them: 1) She showed *compassion* when the lady objected to being artificially fed; 2) She was a key person in the team who had an ability to *communicate* with the lady, not just about her treatment, but also her likes and dislikes and life history; 3) She demonstrated *courage* in advocating on behalf of the lady at multidisciplinary team meetings with senior colleagues; 4) She demonstrated *competence* in encouraging the lady to sip fluids, nibble at food and attend to hygiene/skin care needs; 5) she showed a *commitment* to including patient preferences in the care plan; and 4) She applied principles of sensitive end-of-life *care* in offering comfort and companionship to the lady.
On reflection, what could you have done differently? As far as this patient was concerned, the student felt that she had done the right thing because it was what the lady wanted, and she felt it would have been uncaring to force feed her against her will. Perhaps the student might have considered ways to stimulate the lady's appetite and assess other possible causes of anorexia.
What are you doing to improve decision-making skills? The student was a participant in a research project investigating the development of nurses' clinical decision-making skills. This prompted her to reflect upon and learn from decisions she made.

Table 7.4 Applying 'PERSON' to evaluate clinical decision-making in the 'refusal of treatment' case study

The above example of applying the 'PERSON' evaluation tool to review how a real-life ethical dilemma was dealt with illustrates its potential usefulness as a framework with which to evaluate nurses' clinical decision-making and the quality of care given to patients. Using 'PERSON' will therefore help you to develop and demonstrate the required NMC proficiencies identified at the start of this chapter (Platform 1: Being an accountable professional; Platform 2: Promoting health and preventing ill health; Platform 3: Assessing and planning care; Platform 4: Providing and evaluating care; and Platform 6: Improving safety and quality of care).

Activity 7.11 Reflection

The importance of achieving the proficiency 6.7 'Improving safety and quality of care' (NMC, 2018a) listed at the start of this chapter reflects the findings of the Francis Report (2013) into poor standards of practice. One of its main recommendations was for health professionals to exercise 'a duty of candour', which means to be open, honest and transparent about the quality of care that patients receive, and to take action to address any concerns that patients, relatives, carers or other service users may have. It is therefore important that you are able to demonstrate an ability to critically evaluate the care you give. Please use the 'PERSON' evaluation tool as a framework to evaluate patient care that you have contributed to.

As this is based on your own reflections, there is no outline answer at the end of the chapter.

Chapter summary

This chapter has described ten perceptions of clinical decision-making in nursing (collaborative; experience and intuition; confidence; systematic; prioritising; observation; standardised; reflective; ethical sensitivity; accountability) derived from researching nursing students' development of decision-making skills over a four-year period from beginning their nursing programme to their first year as registered nurses. The ten perceptions of clinical decision-making were related to, and shown to complement, the different kinds of evidence influencing practice and dispositions of the evidence-based nurse (described in Chapter 1). Case studies and scenarios from different nursing pathways were presented, giving a context to explore the application of clinical decision-making skills in evidence-based nursing. A high level of patient contact gives nurses many decision-making opportunities regarding planned care, unplanned 'on-the-spot' responses and contingency plans applied in emergency situations. Sometimes mistakes are made and patients receive poor care. Hence, it is important to evaluate and take action to improve the quality of care. A 'PERSON' evaluation tool was presented to evaluate clinical decision-making in evidence-based nursing. It is recommended as a useful framework for you to evaluate your clinical decision-making and to demonstrate your commitment in achieving high standards of patient-centred evidence-based nursing.

Activities: Brief outline answers

Activity 7.1 Critical thinking (page 129)

Dispositions of the evidence-based nurse	Perceptions of clinical decision-making relating to the dispositions	Examples in the case study of linking the dispositions and perceptions
Other regarding	Collaborative, observation	Supporting the patient's wife, communicating with the theatre team.

(Continued)

Dispositions of the evidence-based nurse	Perceptions of clinical decision-making relating to the dispositions	Examples in the case study of linking the dispositions and perceptions
Engaged with self	Experience and intuition, confidence	Use of self to make a difference in caring for others.
Questioning	Prioritising, systematic	Assessing that there was time to address the patient's wife's needs.
Reflective	Reflective, observation	Judging that offering the wife support in this way was appropriate.
Reflexive	Accountability, reflective	Evaluating effectiveness of care using the patient's wife's feedback.
Creative thinker	Experience and intuition, reflective	Enabling the wife to go to the theatre and creating space for her to talk.
Critical thinker	Systematic, standardised	Applying the principles of therapeutic communication with the patient's wife.
Morally active	Ethical sensitivity, collaborative	Recognising and acting on a duty of care to the patient's wife.

Activity 7.2 Reflection (page 130)

In reflecting on whether the ten identified perceptions of clinical decision-making skills apply equally to planned versus unplanned decisions, you may have concluded as follows:

- All ten perceptions may apply to both planned and unplanned decisions.
- Standardised decisions more closely relate to planned nursing care, but there is also a standardised option to deal with unplanned situations that you don't feel competent to deal with – that is, to get help from an experienced nurse to maximise safe outcomes for patients.
- Experience and intuition more closely relate to unplanned nursing care, but it is also useful to develop intuitive senses in judging whether planned care really suits individual patients.

Activity 7.3 Research and finding out (page 131)

In reflecting on whether any of the ten perceptions of clinical decision-making skills should be applied in all situations (planned, unplanned or emergency), you may have identified:

- accountability – as all decisions have to be justifiable and defensible;
- ethical sensitivity – as all decisions should be in patients' best interests;
- observation – to accurately assess patients and evaluate outcomes of care;
- prioritising – to identify and control perceived risks to patients' well-being.

Activity 7.5 Decision-making (page 135)

In applying the Activities of Living model to do a risk assessment of, and to manage someone having, a generalised tonic-clonic epileptic seizure (fit) you may have identified the following:

- maintaining a safe environment – remove objects or furniture that may cause injury;
- communicating – assure person that someone will stay with them to ensure that they are safe;
- breathing – loosen collar, place the person on side to prevent tongue obstructing airway;
- eating and drinking – remove food from mouth where necessary to prevent choking;

- eliminating – understand that the person may be incontinent during the seizure;
- personal cleansing and dressing – enable person to wash/change clothes afterwards if needed;
- controlling body temperature – adjust clothing/room ventilation to assist temperature control;
- mobilising – loss of voluntary movement, so minimise injury from involuntary muscle spasms;
- working and playing – help person to manage epilepsy so that they can get on with their life;
- expressing sexuality – person may feel self-conscious or undignified and in need of privacy;
- sleeping – person may need to sleep afterwards; if so, it is safer for them to remain on their side;
- preparing for dying – any seizure increases health risks, but a series of repeated generalised tonic-clonic seizures is a life-threatening condition (status epilepticus) requiring urgent medical intervention.

Activity 7.9 Reflection (page 141)

In reflecting on whether the night nurse could have been more vigilant, whether he was negligent and the evidence that could have helped alert him of the risk, you might have said the following:

- Yes, he could have been more vigilant as it is never acceptable to lose a patient.
- No, he was not negligent as his actions were reasonable in the circumstances.
- The most important source of evidence for the new night nurse would have been the verbal information received in the handover. For example, he should have been told if the young man required constant observation and then he would have been able to prioritise his care.

Further reading

Ellis, P, Standing, M and Roberts, S (2020) *Patient Assessment and Care Planning in Nursing* (3rd edn). London: Sage/Learning Matters.

Chapter 10 has a worked example of the 'PERSON' evaluation tool applied to patient assessment decisions.

Standing, M (2020) *Clinical Judgement and Decision-Making in Nursing* (4th edn). London: Sage/Learning Matters.

Explores and applies ten perceptions of decision-making skills in detail. Introduces and critiques a 'PERSON' evaluation tool with which to evaluate clinical decision-making and nursing care.

Useful websites

www.careopinion.org.uk

Encourages patients to say what they liked or did not like about care received to inform other patients about healthcare services (also useful for nurses and other healthcare workers to reflect on their clinical decision-making).

www.nice.org.uk

National Institute for Health and Care Excellence website in which you can search for evidence-based guidelines for many different procedures and clinical areas.

www.nmc.org.uk/concerns-nurses-midwives/hearings/hearings-sanctions/

NMC website link to fitness to practise hearings within previous three months. Select a month from left of screen to see the list of hearings, scroll down end column 'Outcome and reasons' and click to see summary of charges and details of any sanctions imposed.

Chapter 8 Using evidence in the workplace

Peter Ellis

4.1 demonstrate and apply an understanding of what is important to people and how to use this knowledge to ensure their needs for safety, dignity, privacy, comfort and sleep can be met, acting as a role model for others in providing evidence based person-centred care.

4.2 work in partnership with people to encourage shared decision making in order to support individuals, their families and carers to manage their own care when appropriate.

Platform 5: Leading and managing nursing care and working in teams

At the point of registration, the registered nurse will be able to:

5.1 understand the principles of effective leadership, management, group and organisational dynamics and culture and apply these to team working and decision-making.

5.12 understand the mechanisms that can be used to influence organisational change and public policy, demonstrating the development of political awareness and skills.

Chapter aims

After reading this chapter, you will be able to:

- explain why the adoption and implementation of evidence is important;
- demonstrate awareness of some of the barriers to adopting evidence in nursing practice;
- identify strategies for implementing change at the team and organisational level;
- engage in strategies for self-development as an evidence-based nurse.

Introduction

So far, this book has identified a number of sources and types of knowledge and evidence, as well as ways of looking at and applying the evidence to clinical decision-making. Knowledge and evidence are in themselves only conceptual entities; nursing, however, is a practical undertaking and it is important therefore that knowledge and evidence are translated into the practice of nursing. This chapter considers how we might become more evidence-based in our individual and team practice – how we get evidence into the workplace.

Getting evidence, of whatever form, into practice is not as easy as using information we know to have been tested to inform our everyday nursing practice. Before new evidence is adopted, there is a clear need for nurses to assess what is already done in practice and how good its outcomes are – we need to establish what we already know.

Once we understand what we already know and what we already do, and once new evidence has been identified, its quality checked and its suitability for practice established, the next step is to understand what needs to be done in order to get it into practice.

In conjunction with thinking about the steps that must be taken for a new practice to be adopted, it is important to work out what might constitute barriers to its implementation.

Kitson et al. (1998) identify that evidence is most successfully adopted into practice when the evidence is scientifically robust, it mirrors what professionals think and it is in line with patient preferences. As well as these issues, NICE (2018) suggest that the culture of care has to be one that is accepting of change and where there is effective leadership, as well as a willingness to work with others in place. But this is not the whole story; in their research into how national guidelines are negotiated and adopted, Sundberg et al. (2017) identified that in reality people make compromises between rigour and pragmatism – that is to say, that while there may be hard scientific evidence for a particular approach, in the real world people have to consider what will realistically work.

This chapter will explore some of the psychosocial and practical barriers to the adoption of new evidence. It will explore what might need to be done by individuals and teams to facilitate the successful adoption of new ways of working. The potential benefits of adopting evidence in practice from the point of view of the individual practitioner, the team and, importantly, the patient will also be examined.

A model of the dispositions and influences on the evidence-based nurse was advanced in Chapter 1 (Figure 1.1, p24). This model suggests that any nurse who wishes to act in an evidence-based manner needs to engage with certain behaviours and ways of enquiring, all of which are complementary and supplementary to each other.

Activity 8.1   Reflection

Revisit Activity 1.7 on p23, which asked you to explore your understanding of your own existing dispositions, as well as the reasons why you are in nursing. Now that you have read more of the book and have thought about the messages it contains, do you think that any of your identified dispositions or influences are helpful, or unhelpful, to adopting an evidence-based approach to practice?

As this activity is based on your own observations, there is no outline answer at the end of the chapter.

Clearly, the adoption of evidence for practice has been at the heart of this book. Throughout the chapter, you should try to bear in mind that we have so far identified many sources of potential evidence for practice and that the adoption of this evidence will draw on all of these sources to differing degrees at different times.

Questions to ask before adopting new evidence

We have already established that not all information constitutes evidence because it needs to be assessed for its quality before it can be considered as knowledge fit for practice. As well as assessing the sources and quality of the evidence, it is also necessary to consider how well it aligns with clinical need, resources and skills available, how the workplace is organised and managed, and, most importantly, the needs of the clients to whom, and with whom, the evidence will be applied.

These important issues help to ground the adoption of evidence in the realities of practical nursing. Evidence-based practice for nursing is about dealing judiciously with the sources and complexities of knowledge with one foot firmly in the theoretical camp and the other firmly rooted in practice.

Some theorists claim that nursing is an art and others that it is a science. Certainly, there are elements of both philosophies within nursing practice. If the science of nursing is about understanding the biological and physical aspects of care, perhaps the art of nursing is the ability to draw upon multiple and varied strands of knowledge in pursuit of the best holistic outcomes for our patients.

The activity of nursing is unique because of what it does and the people who do it. What nurses do is varied and tends to be whatever needs to be done. This ability to see the big picture and act upon it (being holistic) and to know where to go to get help to achieve this goal (see the discussion on interprofessional practice in Chapter 6) is what sets nursing apart from many other more specialist care professions. Few other professions can truly claim to stand with the patient at the heart of care (being person-centred), displaying humanity and humility, while simultaneously interacting with other professions to achieve good care outcomes (collaborating interprofessionally). The potential for achieving this uniqueness relies heavily on the dispositions and abilities of the individual nurse. It is a potential that becoming evidential, in the broad sense we have demonstrated in this book, can allow us to achieve.

One of the first challenges for nurses attempting to adopt new evidence is identifying and overcoming the real (and understandable if not always acceptable) barriers to change.

Barriers to getting evidence into practice

There are a number of barriers to the adoption of evidence, involving a mix of rational and less rational fears and anxieties. Many of us like to return to places and practices with which we are familiar, things and ideas that reside within our comfort zones. Others are always up for change and challenge, regarding the new and unknown as something to be embraced.

Concept summary: personality types

In one of the most frequently referred to models of the adoption of innovation, Rogers (1962) asserts that there are five different personality types.

- *Innovators* The first 2.5 per cent of adopters are educated, adventurous and risk takers.
- *Early adopters* The next 13.5 per cent are social leaders, popular and educated.
- *Early majority* The next 34 per cent are deliberate and motivated by evolutionary changes.
- *Late majority* The next 34 per cent are sceptical and more traditional.
- *Laggards* The last 16 per cent are technology sceptics who tend not to believe that technology can enhance productivity.

When managing our own personal and professional development as well as change in others, we recognise that not everyone shares the same orientations to change. Nurses, like other people, will adopt a stance to change that is based to some extent on the sort of person they are, their previous experiences of change and their belief in the usefulness of the proposed change and the person proposing the change. Barriers to change therefore arise at a personal, experiential and interpersonal level, and we need to consider these barriers to transition and change before attempting to adopt evidence.

Many nurses do not like change because they understand the practices they are used to and they can predict the likely outcomes of the associated activities – for example, when using a well-tried wound dressing, the nurse will understand what a healing wound looks like on changing the dressing, but with a new dressing the look of the wound may differ, even though the progress of the wound's healing is going well.

Change takes energy and when people are already working hard, the energy needed to undertake change can be overwhelming, especially when the benefits of the change are not thought to include reducing the time and effort that people have to put into their work. There is a management mantra which says that all improvement is change, but not all change is improvement; this mantra is readily adopted by people who are resisting change, especially when they cannot see that the change is, in fact, an improvement. Of course, the other interpretation is that to achieve an improvement in care change is necessary.

Some of the reasons people do not like to change what they do are deeply seated in our natural desire to be thought well of. For example, if a nurse who has been practising clinically for 20 years is confronted with the need to change a practice that she or he has engaged with throughout their entire clinical career, a number of questions may arise.

- What is the point of the change when what I do already is good enough?
- If I adopt this change now, am I saying that what I have done to date has not been good enough?

- How do I know that this change will work?
- Do I have the skills to operate in a new way?

These are reasonable questions, all of which may threaten the status and confidence of the nurse confronted by change. These are sensitive issues that threaten to undermine not only one individual, but potentially the stability of the team and thereby impact on patient care. There are some simple, but pertinent, responses to these questions.

Case study: Managing change

Yvette is the manager of a small team of community nurses. She has been charged with introducing a change of dressing used to treat venous leg ulcers for the whole team. The team contains some people who have been in practice for decades and who are resistant to the change because they know what works and don't see why they should change. Yvette has to get them onside by reminding them that what they do changes regularly, as new treatments come along and that this change will improve care based on new knowledge. Yvette also has to reassure them that all that is changing is the dressing; the skills they bring to the process remain the same.

Resistance to change often arises out of a lack of understanding of the need for change. In these instances, individuals cannot see that current practice is potentially not as good as it might be. They may also not appreciate that the effects of the change may outweigh the time and energy required to make the change, and that in the long run the change may benefit both them and their patients. The need to fulfil their current obligations takes precedence over making changes because the 'here and now' is urgent and change takes time and energy (Ellis, 2022b) and many nurses feel that they lack the skills to implement change (Rodgers, 1994).

Case study: Barriers to evidence-based practice in a nursing home

In their study of barriers to introducing resident-centred care in nursing homes, Engle et al. (2017) identified that in low-performing nursing homes, staff identified staffing, resources, acuity of residents, quality of care conflicts and regulations as reasons for not adopting resident-centred care. Additionally, staff in these homes identified administrator turnover and lack of guidance, the home's culture, staff morale and difficulty working with residents and families as reasons that resident-centred care was not adopted. Even in the more resident-centred homes, staff identified that inconsistency across the home was an issue. This research suggests that the barriers to adopting good practice may be cultural, practical and philosophical.

A lack of vision and understanding of the change can stand in the way of individual nurses accepting change. Sometimes this lack of understanding arises out of the inability of a change agent (perhaps a manager or fellow nurse) to adequately explain what they are doing and the likely outcome. There is an issue of communication here that will need to be addressed if change is to be managed at team level.

Often there are issues with the way in which change is rolled out. Some team members may feel that the process of change has been poorly handled – it is too rapid or too slow, or communication could have been better. Others may feel that the change is not something they agree with, or they may consider the evidence underpinning the change is incomplete or needs further scrutiny.

Activity 8.2   Critical thinking

Consider your personal responses to changes in your personal and work life. Consider the sorts of emotions you experience during periods of change and what this says about why you respond to change as you do.

As this activity is based on your own experiences, there is no outline answer at the end of the chapter.

On other occasions, the introduction of new evidence is hard to instigate because team members have experienced poorly managed change and are sceptical about any subsequent changes.

In their synthesis of the qualitative evidence about barriers and facilitators of change in care settings, McArthur et al. (2021) identified a number of barriers to implementing evidence-based guidelines:

- Lack of time.
- Lack of staffing.
- Lack of resources.
- Lack of teamwork.
- Lack of organisational support.
- Practical difficulties with the care environment and culture.
- Lack of knowledge.
- Change fatigue.

As well as the barriers to change, there are a number of practical barriers to the adoption of evidence-based practice that may need addressing. These include the inability to search online databases, a lack of understanding about research, the inability to access research and a preference for seeking guidance from colleagues (Yoder et al., 2022). We help you to address many of these issues in this book, especially in Chapter 2 where we discuss access to bibliographic databases and how to search them effectively.

If we are concerned about improving lives and providing high-quality care, we need to focus on the shared value of care. Even if our personal orientation is to be sceptical about the sources of some of the evidence we have to employ as nurses, we should assess the value of the information on its own merit and on the merit of the values that underpin it.

Consequences of not adopting evidence-based practice for nursing

Poor decisions in nursing can affect the quality of life and, indeed, the very lives of the patients we care for. We have identified various sources of information and a number of ways of checking the quality of the information before we accept it as evidence. It is now worth asking the question, 'What are the consequences of not adopting an evidential approach to our nursing practice?'

Activity 8.3   Critical thinking

Before you go on to read the next section of this chapter, take a few moments to jot down what you think might be some of the consequences of *not* adopting an evidence-based approach to nursing practice. For example, what might have been the consequences of failing to evaluate effectiveness of PPE during the height of the pandemic? When doing this, think about the consequences for patients as well as nurses and nursing in general.

An outline answer is provided at the end of the chapter.

Internationally, nursing is still creating and consolidating its professional identity. One of the characteristics of a profession is that it has its own body of knowledge which establishes its credentials and credibility within society. Adopting the broad approach to evidence advocated in this book goes some way towards establishing this credible knowledge base, creating and enhancing the identity of nursing as a profession in its own right. This book provides a blueprint for establishing the credibility of nursing evidence, while at the same time recognising what is special about nursing as an activity.

If nurses fail to adopt evidential care practices, there will doubtless be consequences for the image of nursing as a whole. It may not immediately be obvious to some why maintaining a positive image for nursing is important. However, when we think about the need for the people we care for to have trust in what we do at times in their lives when they are perhaps at their most vulnerable, the answers present themselves. Care is best provided and best received when there is trust. Maintaining a positive public perception of nursing engenders trust, and this positive image itself derives from nurses being able to demonstrate that their practice is worthwhile.

Within *The Code* for nurses and midwives (NMC, 2018b) there is a requirement for nurses to:

6 Always practise in line with the best available evidence

To achieve this, you must:

6.1 make sure that any information or advice given is evidence-based, including information relating to using any healthcare products or services, and

6.2 maintain the knowledge and skills you need for safe and effective practice.

Regardless of our professional standing, it remains the duty of nurses to communicate effectively, in a manner that can be understood, with our clients and colleagues. The important message here is that when applying evidence we should not neglect our core activities of care and communication. Rather, the application of an evidence base to practice should be used to supplement and complement what we do, as we have seen in the platforms and proficiencies identified at the start of the chapter.

Scholtes (1998), when talking about how to gain trust as a leader, suggests that there are two elements that need to be got right. The first element is that the leader has to demonstrate that he or she has the ability to get the job done and the second is that they care about their staff. If we translate this idea into the evidence-based nursing care scenario, we might readily see trust not only as being a function of the ability to demonstrate care for the people we are nursing, but also as showing that we know what we are doing and why (we have the ability to get the job done).

Failure to act in an evidential manner in our practice therefore puts nurses at odds with the regulations of our registering body and creates questions about fitness to practise. The platforms and proficiencies identified at the start of this chapter require nurses to be competent in care delivery and in the improvement of standards for nursing practice.

Theory

Adopting and adapting to the challenges of evidence-based nursing practice is about the constant improvement of care. Within the context of evidence-based nursing presented in this book, the knowledge underpinning these improvements is regarded as having been judiciously identified, conscientiously analysed and proactively adopted. Reflecting on the content of these statements, it is clear to see why evidence-based nursing care is a realistic and feasible route to fulfilling the requirements of both the NMC *Code* (2018b) and the Standards of Proficiency for Registered Nurses (2018a).

Acting in the best interests of our clients is a desirable attribute of nursing, although it may not always be clear what constitutes best interests (Ellis, 2019, 2020). Whatever view you choose to take of what 'best interests of patients' means, be this improving their health or maintaining their dignity, what is clear is that no patient's best interests can be served in a meaningful way without some understanding of the evidence base underpinning their care. This is not an empty statement since the evidence base of nursing care is concerned not only with what practices serve to make people physically or psychologically better, but also with an understanding of how people experience care.

Accountability

The accountability that trained nurses have for the safety and quality of the care they provide can be demonstrated by the adoption of evidence-based nursing practice. Failure to adopt evidence will mean that nurses cannot justify the care they give (NMC, 2018b). While it is true that the obligations of student nurses do not operate at the level of accountability to the regulatory body, they are responsible for their own actions and omissions in the provision of care, becoming accountable for these on qualifying. It would seem sensible, therefore, to adopt a critical and evidence-based approach to practice sooner rather than later.

Accountability is not merely about how we conduct ourselves in practice; it is also about the things we do. Accountability on this level is being able to justify the tasks we perform using our professional knowledge and skills; such knowledge is drawn down from our understanding of evidence.

As well as our obligations to our profession and its regulatory body, nurses have obligations and duties to their employers. These duties extend to fulfilling our roles as nurses within the clinical governance frameworks established and monitored by our employer and nationally. Clinical governance requirements mean that, as nurses, we need to be able to demonstrate what we do is clinically effective and achieved in a manner which is safe, effective, caring, responsive and well led (Pearson, 2017).

It seems self-evident that the achievement of safe, caring and effective outcomes for patients is best accomplished by nursing staff who can identify, understand and apply evidence to practice.

Moral imperative

Ethically, it is hard to justify the provision of care that is not evidence-based, where evidence exists. There are many occasions when there is little or no apparent *hard* evidence to support what we do as nurses. This does not, however, mean that what is done to, and with, the patient is unethical. It does mean that as well as striving to do the best for the patient (beneficence – Beauchamp and Childress, 2013), the nurse operating as an evidential practitioner takes the time to reflect in and on action, and adds the experiential learning to their own constantly evolving evidence base (see Chapter 5).

There is a moral duty on the part of the nurse to use more objective and rigorous forms of evidence to support their practice, where such evidence exists (NMC, 2018b). This obligation arises out of the special contractual obligations nurses accept on entering the nursing profession. This contract states that we will provide care to the best of our ability and that patients can expect us to do so, not because we are fellow human beings necessarily (although this is also an important factor in establishing our obligations), but because we have taken on and accepted this additional duty of our own free will (Ellis, 2012).

On some occasions nurses may be required to justify the care they have given in a court of law. To this end, it is important that nurses can demonstrate beyond reasonable doubt that they have provided the care they can both realistically and professionally be expected to provide. Unfortunately, litigation against healthcare professionals, including nurses, is increasing; it is therefore both necessary and wise to ensure that our nursing practice is able to stand up to this level of scrutiny.

The main reason that evidence is important is that it improves the quality of the care that nurses undertake (Crabtree et al., 2016). Nurses should, and indeed most do, take pride in what they do, and this pride should stem from an understanding that what they do is the very best they can achieve. Providing good-quality care is both good in its own right (it is a duty), as well as being important because of its consequences (the outcomes for patients; Ellis, 2020). The key consequence of high-quality care that is firmly grounded in critical and evidential nursing practice is that it improves not only the outcomes of care, but also the patient's experience of it.

Activity 8.4   Reflection

Try to remember a time when you were in receipt of nursing or any other form of healthcare. How did you feel about the care given and was this affected by your perception of the person/people giving the care? Why?

An outline answer is provided at the end of the chapter.

Managing change and transition

Change can be considered to be an alteration to the way in which something is done or the replacement of one thing by another. For example, a hospital or department may choose to change the type of dressing they use post-operatively, or a ward may be remodelled in order to be able to achieve the Department of Health's single-sex ward requirement.

Transition is an alteration in the mindset of the people who have to undertake change (Bridges and Bridges, 2017). Regardless of the purpose or nature of a change, all change engenders an emotional and psychological response from those concerned as they have to undergo a transition in their thinking. Before we go on to examine the management of change, both in ourselves and in others, it is worth stopping for a moment to consider the psychological impact of change.

Tools such as the Holmes and Rahe (1967) Social Readjustment Rating Scale identify that any life change is associated with stress, even ones that we want to happen such as starting a new job or getting married. Hopson and Adams (1976) proposed a model that explains the changes in self-esteem that people go through in periods of transition and captures some of the reasons why people might become stressed (see Figure 8.1).

This model of changes in self-esteem during transition demonstrates that there is a level of loss and adjustment associated with all changes. What the model does not show is that the transition through the model is not always the same for all people, or even for any single individual. In fact, Hopson and Adams (1976) claim that different people go through the stages in different orders at different times, and that not everyone goes through every stage for each transition they go through. The stages of transition in the model are defined in Table 8.2.

What these models of the psychological impacts of change and transition tell us is that negative psychological responses are normal. It is important, therefore, that we accept that when we are exposed to change, there will be a psychological response, and this is something we should learn to cope with for ourselves, and recognise and manage in others.

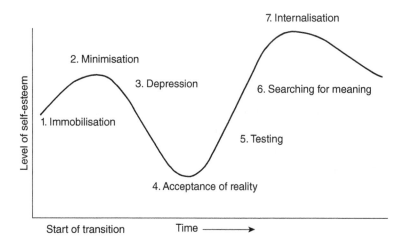

Figure 8.1 A model of changes in self-esteem during transitions, as described by Hopson and Adams (1976)

Immobilisation	A sense of being overwhelmed and unable to act when faced with a transition. Transitions that are unfamiliar and ones that are associated with negative expectations tend to intensify this stage.
Minimisation	A coping mechanism when faced with change. Frequently, people deny the change is happening. This is a common reaction to a crisis which is too difficult to face.
Depression	People may become depressed when faced with the implications of change.
Acceptance of reality	Occurs at the point when people begin to let go of their old state of being and start to accept the reality of the change.
Testing	Begins when the reality of the change has been accepted. In this stage, people start to try out new behaviours to cope with the new situation.
Searching for meaning	A reflective stage during which people try to work out how and why things are different.
Internalisation	The final stage of the process during which understandings of the new situation become accepted. The new understanding then becomes part of the person's behaviour.

Table 8.1 What the stages of the model of changes in self-esteem during transitions mean. Based on the work of Hopson and Adams, 1976.

Managing change and transition as an individual

As identified in the model of evidence-based practice in Chapter 1, nurses who choose to practise as evidence-based practitioners must first engage with themselves. This engagement with self is about understanding our own behaviours and orientations. It is about understanding who we are and why we act as we do. One of the mechanisms for doing this that has been identified in this book is the use of reflection and clinical supervision. It is only by examining what we think and feel about situations we have been in, and experiences we have had, that we can critically reflect upon who we are and what motivates us. Other strategies have included being more aware of the nursing literature, especially research, and engaging in a meaningful way with it.

Becoming evidence-based requires a nurse to make two transitions. The first of these involves accepting that nursing is about being responsive to new sources of knowledge, new evidence and new understandings. We have to accept that this transition is about lifelong learning, and continuing personal and professional development, and that change is an inevitable consequence of working in health and social care; indeed, it is part of the social contract we enter into as we accept the role of a professional caregiver.

The second transition involves learning to work with the various sources of knowledge and evidence identified within this book, and understanding how these separate types of evidence can be worked into a larger scheme of understanding. Internalisation of these realities is fundamental to both becoming, and continuing as, an evidence-based nurse.

Reasons why nurses need to constantly evolve and adapt what they do and engage in lifelong learning include:

- emergence of new diseases and the understanding of disease, e.g. COVID-19;
- development of new treatments;
- changing demographics within society;
- the changing expectations of patients;
- increasing professionalisation of nursing;
- increasing understanding of the impacts of care.

So, what does this mean for you as an individual student or qualified nurse? There is a real challenge here in that understanding yourself as a nurse will have a direct impact on how you see yourself as a person. Undoubtedly, reflection – trying to make sense of situations and planning how you will act in the future (Jasper, 2013) – and reflexivity – awareness of yourself and your impact on the working environment (Esterhuizen, 2019) – are skills that are absolutely necessary to function effectively as a nurse in today's care environments. Employing reflection and reflexivity are essential for consolidating the skills and knowledge that you currently have, as well as identifying what skills and knowledge you need to develop.

What is clear from this message is that doing nothing is not really an option for nurses who wish to be both patient-centred and evidence-based. The messages contained in this book point to the need to integrate into our understanding of care not only our own reflections, but also the views of our patients and insights from our colleagues.

Activity 8.5   Research and finding out

As you embark on the start of your career as a nurse, now is the time to establish some good habits about how you will continue to grow and develop as a nurse. Identify the strategies you can put in place to ensure that you remain both a lifelong learner and evidential in your practice. Create a personal development plan for achieving these.

An outline answer is provided at the end of the chapter.

Critical and creative thinking

Critical and creative thinking, as well as reflection and reflexivity, can be used to enhance both self-development and practice. The skills necessary for criticality and creativity are different, but also complementary, and both enhance the ability of the nurse to become an evidence-based practitioner.

We identified in our model of evidence-based practice in Chapter 1 that creative and critical thinking are dispositions of the evidence-based nurse. Throughout the book we have seen examples of creative and critical thinking under different guises in the identification of sources of evidence, in the processing (critiquing) of evidence and, finally, in the adoption of evidence. But what are creative and critical thinking, and how might they help us become more evidence-based practitioners?

Critical thinking

Being a critical thinker requires that we adopt the disposition of being inquisitive and receptive to new forms and sources of knowledge. It also requires that this inquisitiveness is guided by an inquisitive attitude and well-honed strategic skills (Falcó-Pegueroles, 2021). This means enquiry that is both conscious (we choose to do it) and conscientious (we follow a well-defined pattern of thought) and is arguably a virtue (Falcó-Pegueroles, 2021). Hence, critical thinking is about clarity and rationality of thought.

As critical thinking involves clarity and rationality, it can help lead the nurse from being overwhelmed with information to a position where they are able to logically analyse and unite ideas from a number of sources into ideas (or evidence) that are fit for both implementation and further analysis. The need for further analysis arises out of the questioning disposition that we identified in the evidence-based nursing model in Chapter 1, and the realisation that healthcare is constantly evolving and therefore our evidence base and understanding of care need to evolve with it.

Activity 8.6 Critical thinking

Consider how your understanding of nursing has evolved, perhaps because of what you have read, learnt in the classroom or seen in practice. Think about what things you used to find hard to understand – for example, why there is a theory–practice gap – and then consider what you know about these issues now and if it makes more sense now that you have had time to study evidence-based practice.

There are some thoughts and possible answers at the end of the chapter.

Certainly, the notion of the need for constant and repeated analysis through reflexivity and reflection echoes one of the core messages of this book: that knowledge is only knowledge until some new knowledge comes along. This underlines the need for engagement in lifelong learning and continuous personal and professional development. Evidently, critical thinking is not about the accumulation of knowledge, nor is criticality about being argumentative. It is about strategies that enable us to strengthen and deepen our understandings, and develop ideas and theories with which to underpin practice.

So how can we develop as critical thinkers? First of all, we need to take time to look for and understand the logical connections between ideas. For example, we are frequently told that information giving helps reduce stress in our patients, but have we ever thought about why? Many of us know that stress can arise out of a feeling of loss of control. A feeling of loss of control can arise from not knowing what is happening. So spending time explaining things to patients means that they know what is going on, they can make some choices; they feel more in control and therefore less stressed. Next time a patient is angry or irritated by the care they receive, do not jump to the conclusion they are being rude – ask yourself why. This is critical thinking.

Concept summary: Empiricism

Empiricism is based on two related ideas: the first is that all knowledge stems from things we can experience with our senses; it also maintains a place for the sorts of knowledge that arise through research and experimentation. The second key idea of empiricism is that all knowledge is tentative – that is, knowledge is only knowledge until a new way of understanding something supersedes it.

In much the same way, we can solve all manner of problems by thinking clearly and logically, looking for connections between ideas and theories of knowledge that enable us to make sense of what is happening.

Critical thinking is therefore about honing our understanding of an issue by systematically bringing together threads of an argument in a logical way in order to solve problems or create new understandings (Jackson and Ellis, 2010). A useful metaphor is that critical thinking acts like a funnel, collecting lots of diverse information and knowledge, and narrowing it down to something more manageable (evidence).

Creative thinking

For the evidence-based practitioner, creativity follows on logically from criticality. Once we have thought about and understood something, we can decide how we might use the new learning in our practice; sometimes this requires us to be creative. Creative thinking is about exploring possibilities, creating solutions and generating new ideas and ways of moving practice forward (Smith et al., 2014). Evidently, if we have engaged in critical thinking and thereby understood a situation or scenario, then as an evidence-based nurse grounded in action, we need to generate ideas about how we are going to act. Creative thinking therefore feeds into the idea of change and transition.

If we pick up the funnel metaphor once more, while critical thinking narrows a lot of diverse information and knowledge together into evidence, creative thinking may be thought of as more like an inverted funnel, taking the evidence and placing it in among issues such as existing policy, professional and patient preference, ethical considerations and practical knowledge. This broadening out in thinking allows realistic and practical considerations to be made about the application of the evidence to practice (Jackson and Ellis, 2010).

Creativity is, therefore, the ability to generate new ways of thinking and/or working. This ability arises out of conscientious exploration of sources of evidence and critical appraisal of their worth. Creativity is also an attitude – a 'can do' attitude that says, 'There is an issue here where my knowledge and the realities of this situation do not marry up. I will therefore find a way to make sense of this situation.' Being creative is a process in which we constantly seek to refine and enhance what we do, taking into account a broader perspective on practice.

Having engaged in critical thinking activities that identify problems and sources of evidence, we can then use creativity either to solve problems or to improve on what we do. The key to creative thinking is the understanding that there might be more than one solution to an issue that is correct, and that the solutions to a problem might vary according to the situation, resources available and the people involved.

This idea of the contextual reality of creativity marries well with the central theme of this book. The reality of providing evidential person-centred care requires us to engage with other nurses, other care professionals, other agencies and, most importantly, with the patient, their family and other carers. Engaging with others allows us to see a clinical scenario from more than one viewpoint; it demonstrates the multiplicity of reality and the fact that each episode of care, while often following similar trajectories, is unique.

Being open to critical and creative thinking, therefore, develops the ability within us to adapt our way of thinking and adopt new practices in care. It allows us to deal with change and transition in a proactive and managed way, and generates for the individual the ability to be truly evidence-based.

Managing change and transition in teams

So far in this chapter, we have laid out some challenges and solutions to becoming an evidence-based practitioner. In this section we will take the ideas one step further and explore how we might manage the process of change and transition in the team setting.

Getting evidence into practice in a team is all about the management of change, and sustaining the impetus of change management is all about creating environments of care that are not only responsive to evidence, but are also environments in which nurses and other care professionals actively seek out opportunities to incorporate evidence into their day-to-day practice.

Tamunomiebi and Uhuru (2018) argue that teams exist to get a job done. Meeting the needs of patients requires nurses to take account of not only the roles of the members of their immediate team, but also those of the extended interprofessional team, other teams and agencies and, importantly, the needs of the patients (Elliott and Koubel, 2009).

Lewin's (1947) model of change is often cited in management training. It is a simple model that reflects many of the aspects of change that need to be accounted for if change is to be managed successfully.

Lewin's model is called 'the freeze, unfreeze, freeze model', and is perhaps best thought of by thinking about a block of ice. If you want to change a block of ice from a cube shape to a sphere, then the best way to change it is to first unfreeze it, and then (while it is liquid) pour it into a new mould before freezing it again. This approach is in preference to the 'chip bits off until you get the required shape', which is both time-consuming and subject to inaccuracy in the final result (Ellis and Abbott, 2018).

Similarly, if you want to instigate change in people, you must find a way to get them from where they are now (the initial freeze stage) to where you want them to be by getting them to 'unfreeze' the way they think and behave, to adapt to a new perspective and then freeze again in the new way of behaving or thinking. To complete the metaphor, this is better than wearing people down in an attempt to achieve the desired change, which is both time-consuming and may not achieve the desired effect.

What, then, does this tell us about how to get evidence-based changes adopted by the teams or organisations in which we work? First, there is the issue of identifying what we do now and why (the initial freeze). This allows us to explore the quality of what we do. In order to change, we need to decide what it is we want to change, why and how.

This first stage is all about communication and setting the vision for how things might be and what outcomes we might expect if we decide to change (Bridges and Bridges, 2017). One example might be the introduction of a new pressure ulcer dressing in the general ward. First, we might undertake an audit of the use of such dressings now. This audit might include quantifying how many dressings we use, how much each dressing costs, how frequently the dressing has to be changed, how easy the dressing is to use, the effectiveness of the dressing (how long a particular grade of ulcer takes to heal), the acceptability of the dressing to the patient, the incidence of infection in patients using the dressing and any associated costs of cleansing the wound. This information provides benchmarking data against which we might trial a new dressing.

We may then decide that we want to speed up the process of healing or reduce the incidence of infection-related complications in patients with similar ulcers. A review of the literature on pressure ulcers and discussions with experienced and expert staff in wound management might then be used to understand the options available. Some understanding of the pros and cons of the new approach and some ideas about exactly what it is that we want to achieve will create the vision for how things might be. During this stage, it is important to engage all the team in the process so they know what the purpose of the change is and can contribute ideas and insights, as well as discuss fears and potential barriers.

During the initial planning stage, strategies such as education, clinical supervision, team meetings and management support might be helpful in overcoming resistance (Byers, 2017). These strategies also promote inclusivity and demonstrate a commitment to being 'other regarding', as well as exploiting the potential benefits of working with others.

The process of trialling the change – again, collecting data on the variables identified earlier – is the 'unfreezing' stage. 'Unfreezing' is about trying the alternatives and exploring what advantages might be gained and what problems might arise. Again, it is important to include all the team, as they will then be able to contribute to the evaluation of the change. Failure to include the team can create mistrust and fear; it may lead to some people doing things in a different way from everyone else and can derail the whole process.

As ever, the role of the patient in this process is very important. We cannot know how comfortable the dressing is when in place or how much discomfort is associated with changing it unless we ask. Not only does this allow us to assess another one of our criteria for adopting the change, it again demonstrates a willingness to be 'other regarding' as identified in the dispositions of the evidence-based nurse in Chapter 1.

The move to consolidating practice (the second 'freeze') can then occur when the change has been assessed. It is worthy of note that not all potential evidence-based changes to practice can, or are, adopted in practice because of local issues, such as workload, resistance to change (Moule, 2021) or applicability (Parahoo, 2014).

For the evidence-based nurse, there is little to be gained from going it alone with a change in practice. The benefits that might accrue from advancing and developing practice can only be fully realised if they are adopted by the whole team (see Table 8.2).

Define the need	Quantify use, cost, frequency of changes needed, healing times, incidence of infection. Establish ease of use and patient preference.
Plan ahead	Review the literature. Consult the experts. Define what a good outcome might look like.
Involve the team	Use team meetings. Consider clinical supervision. Use the expertise in the team. Provide education and training.
Trial the new product	Involve all the team. Get feedback on ease of use and patient preference and tolerability.
Assess the feedback	Decide as a team if the change is worth making.
Evaluate practice	Make the change or stick with what you have; evaluate the feeling of the team and move towards establishing the new or re-establishing the old practice.

Table 8.2 Managing the process of changing the choice of dressing.

Any group of individuals who wish to adopt a 'can do' attitude to the delivery of care must develop together. Developing together is about learning together. Teams that learn together and develop their practice from this learning are said to operate in a 'learning culture' (Kamel and Arif, 2017). Teams that operate in a learning culture seek out and embrace the challenges that change brings. Learning cultures become established when staff commit to lifelong learning; such a culture enables teams to thrive in rapidly evolving environments of care where being evidential allows them to become better responsive to, or even producers of, change and innovation. We saw dozens of examples of this during the COVID-19 pandemic, where clinical teams had to quickly adapt time and time again to implement new knowledge about the virus and the ways of preventing onward transmission and treating those affected. Cultures develop in response to the actions of individuals within a team, and therefore the evidence-based nurse is well placed to influence the development and maintenance of a general culture of enquiry and learning, even when he or she occupies a lowly position in said team.

Benefits to the patient

It seems only right to end this book with some thoughts about how evidence-based practice can benefit patients. Throughout the book, we have seen that evidence is not merely about the blind adoption of changes to practice identified from within research papers. We have seen that our own experience, the shared experiences of others and research serve as sources of evidence, and that working with others, reflection, the ability to critique research and a conscientious clinical decision-making process help us to process information into something that informs care. We have also noted at various points along the way that the purpose of adopting an evidential approach to nursing care is not merely about ticking academic or regulatory boxes; it is about benefitting our patients.

What is clear is the evidence-based nurse who takes account of the dispositions and influences on practice identified in the model in Chapter 1 will operate in a way that benefits patients in two important ways.

The first is by including them in the process of generating the evidence base – that is to say, taking account of their experience and knowledge. As well as paying attention to the patient's experience, the evidence-based nurse will also be patient-centred in the decision-making process, taking account of patient preference and perceived need as well as other forms of knowledge.

The second benefit to the patient is perhaps more obvious in that evidence-based nursing care is good-quality care – it is care grounded in carefully generated knowledge. High-quality, acceptable, person-centred care is, after all, what we should all be aiming for.

Chapter summary

The process of getting evidence into practice is one of managing change and transition. Reasons for adopting evidence in practice include improving what we do and how we do it. There are also good moral and ethical imperatives for doing the best we can for patients.

In this chapter we have explored some of the strategies we can use individually and collectively to implement change in the clinical setting. The fundamental purpose for the identification and adoption of evidence is quite simply the improvement of practice.

Throughout the book we have presented a series of challenges to becoming evidence based, and identified a number of strategies and an overall framework that will support the development of this.

Activities: Brief outline answers

Activity 8.3 Critical thinking (page 159)

Failure to adopt an evidential approach to nursing practice will lead to a number of detrimental consequences, some of which are listed here:

- nurse acting under the authority of others rather than autonomously;
- a poor public perception of nursing;
- job dissatisfaction;
- poor use of resources;
- poor outcomes for patients;
- inability to justify what we do and how we do it;
- failure to follow our professional code;
- inability to meet the governance agenda in hospitals.

Activity 8.4 Reflection (page 162)

It is likely that the perceptions of many of us about the people who care for us are based on the impressions we form of them as individuals. This perception will be formed on the basis of their appearance, how they talk to us and who they are. As with all healthcare professionals, the public perception of who they are is based not only on face-to-face meetings, but also on their portrayal in the media. This media image is, at least in part, driven by the scandals and other negative events that occur (for examples, search for the Winterbourne View Abuse Scandal and Report of the Mid Staffordshire NHS Foundation Trust Public Inquiry). There are numerous other examples where the competence of nursing staff to deliver care and recognise abuse, and standards of personal and professional conduct have made the headlines (see Chapter 7); these most certainly impact on the image of the profession as a whole. There is little doubt that some of these issues of competence and behaviour are linked to the lack of commitment of some individuals to provide high-quality evidence-informed care.

Activity 8.5 Research and finding out (page 165)

There are many simple personal strategies that can improve your ability to function as an evidence-based nurse. These strategies include identifying simple sources of evidence you can use to inform your practice. You might, for example, set up e-mail alerts from some of the many nursing and medical websites that provide updates of the most recent articles and research in the area in which you work; you might subscribe to a nursing journal; better still, you might start or join a journal club. Clinical supervision is a powerful tool for self-development, as is engaging in focused conversations about care with your clinical mentor. Service users (patients) provide a great source of insight into how care is experienced and what it is like to be ill. Perhaps you might keep a reflective diary that allows you not only to put on paper what you are thinking and feeling, but to focus on developing the above strategies to enhance your practice.

Activity 8.6 Critical thinking (page 166)

Critical thinking often arises out of repeated exposure to things. This exposure allows us to start to see connections between issues as well as to explore our thinking and feelings. The theory–practice gap can be a devastating realisation for novice nurses who see it as immoral and illogical. Experience and education enable us to reflect on some of the reasons for it, which include many of the barriers to change we have already identified. This process of realisation speeds up as we start to form theories and understanding of reality and start to see the bigger picture and where things fit into this bigger picture. Applying ourselves to thinking about and understanding our realities is critical thinking; it helps us identify why things occur and place them in a greater scheme of understanding and realisation.

Further reading

Ellis, P (2022b) *Leadership, Management and Team Working in Nursing* (4th edn). London: Sage.

See especially Chapter 7 on change management.

Gopee, N and Galloway, J (2017) *Leadership and Management in Healthcare* (3rd edn). London: Sage.

See especially Chapter 6 on leading and managing change.

McCormack, B and McCance, T (2016) *Person-Centred Practice in Nursing and Health Care: Theory and Practice* (2nd edn). Chichester: Wiley-Blackwell.

See especially section 3 – Developing person-centred cultures: A practice development approach.

Price, B (2021) *Critical Thinking and Writing for Nursing Students* (4th edn). London: Sage.

A book for student nurses on how to think critically.

Useful websites

www.businessballs.com/change-management/

A management theory website with some accessible ideas on change management.

www.cqc.org.uk

The Care Quality Commission; look especially at the standards by which services are audited.

www.evidentlycochrane.net/

An evidence-based practice blog site.

www.mindtools.com/pages/article/newTCS_82.htm

Find an explanation of the Holmes and Rahe Stress Scale here.

www.nice.org.uk

The website of the National Institute for Health and Care Excellence.

www.nmc.org.uk

Nursing and Midwifery Council (NMC) website where *The Code* can be found.

https://s4be.cochrane.org/

Students for best evidence is an evidence-based practice resource site for students. See especially the resources page.

Appendix
A generic research critiquing framework with additional paradigm specific questions

The first section of this framework can be applied to all forms of research. The later sections apply specifically to qualitative and quantitative research, and ask questions in a manner specific to these methodologies.

Questions that apply to all research

Background issues

Title

Does this identify:

- the type of people to whom the research is being applied?
- the research question/aims/hypothesis?
- the paradigm/methodology/data-collection method(s)?
- the main finding(s) of the study?

Author credentials

Can you identify the author(s)':

- qualifications?
- professional background?
- current job?
- experience of doing similar research?
- conflicts of interest?

Core research issues

The question

- Does the introduction and background to the study identify the need for the research to be done?
- Can you identify the purpose of the research (its aim(s), question(s) or hypothesis/es)?

Methodology, methods and sampling

- Given the question, do the research paradigm and methodology chosen make sense?
- Even if 'yes', are there alternative methodologies that might also be appropriate?
- Given the methodology identified (if any), are the research data-collection methods correct?
- Even if 'yes', are there alternative methods that might also be appropriate?
- With regard to the sample:
  - Is the method of recruiting identified and reasonable?
  - Might the recruitment method introduce some form of bias?
  - Is the sample of the right size?
  - Do the author(s) discuss how the sample size was calculated/arrived at?
  - Does the sample represent the people the study is about?
  - Even if 'yes', are there alternative strategies that might have made the process as good or better?

Results, conclusions and discussion

- Is the approach to analysis of results consistent with the type of data collected?
- With regard to the results:
  - Is it apparent how the data were analysed?
  - Are these clear?
  - Do they reflect what the researchers set out to answer?
- Does the discussion:
  - reflect the results?
  - reflect the purpose of the research?
  - identify practical issues that have impaired the research?
  - identify compromises that have been made to allow the research to proceed?
  - only make claims about things the research set out to answer?
  - explain why the results have occurred?
  - contain additional results?
- Does the conclusion:
  - only discuss what the aim(s) of the research were about?
  - reflect the results and discussion?
  - identify and compare the results with similar research?
  - identify and compare the results to existing and potential policy?
  - suggest possibilities for future research?

Ethical issues

Have the researchers:

- demonstrated that the research is necessary?
- gained ethics approval?
- demonstrated concern for confidentiality and anonymity?
- shown concern for informed consent including:
    - freedom from coercion (or appearance of potential coercion);
    - information giving;
    - freedom of choice;
    - right of participants to withdraw;
    - extra concern for potentially vulnerable participants?
- Have the researchers shown concern for the ethical principles of:
    - doing good?
    - avoiding unnecessary harm?
    - respecting participant autonomy (see also consent)?
    - respect for fairness?

Additional questions that apply to qualitative research

When critiquing qualitative research, these additional questions, using terms specific to qualitative research, *must* also be considered.

Rigour

- Has the research process been fully explained in a transparent manner that is clear from the article?

Dependability

- Has the study been undertaken in a consistent manner?
- Have all researchers used the same procedures?

Credibility

- Have the researchers checked the level of agreement with their findings – i.e. with more than one person analysing?
- Did the researchers check their interpretation with the participants and/or other professionals?

Confirmability

- Have the data been dealt with in a neutral manner?
- Is the way that the data has been handled clear – auditable?

Transferability

- Does other research appear to support the findings?
- If no, are the reasons for the difference explained coherently?

Additional questions that apply to quantitative research

When critiquing quantitative research, these additional questions, using terms specific to quantitative research, *must* also be considered.

Bias

Have the researchers identified and dealt with potential bias within the study design and execution? Specific biases may include:

- **behavioural bias**;
- measurement bias;
- recall bias;
- response bias;
- sampling bias;
- selection bias.

Confounding

- Are there alternative explanations for what has occurred in the study?

Validity

- Does the study measure what it says it will measure and do the data-collection tools do what they say they do?

Reliability

- Have the researchers demonstrated that the data collection has occurred in a consistent and reproducible manner?

Generalisability and representativeness

- Where the researchers have claimed the study is generalisable, is the study sample representative of the people they claim the findings apply to?

Glossary

action learning set: a structured group-led approach to problem solving by examining scenarios and discussing solutions.

anonymity: the process of protecting or hiding an individual's true identity.

assent: a term often used to denote consent given for another person – e.g., a wife for a husband with dementia.

autonomy: the freedom, and in some senses the ability, to choose what we will do with our lives and our bodies. It implies freedom from pressure from others.

behavioural bias: bias that occurs when people within a study behave in a given manner because of some underlying reason that usually affects all similar individuals.

beneficence: the ethical principle of doing good.

bias: in the context of research, anything in the design or undertaking of a study that causes an untruth to occur in the study, potentially affecting the outcome of the study.

biographic research: research based on the accounts of individuals who have experienced a particular life event, recounted primarily in their own words.

capacity: relates to the ability of an individual to understand information given in the consent process.

case study: a study that explores individual or small, similar accounts of a phenomenon or disease, and may be either quantitative or qualitative.

cathartic interventions: verbal and non-verbal skills enabling others to express feelings.

clinical decision-making: applying clinical judgement to select the best possible evidence-based option to control risks and address patients' needs in order to provide high-quality care, for which you are accountable.

clinical governance: a system of audit and other checks that health services use to check on and improve their services.

cognitively: refers to the ability to be able to think rationally and provide meaning.

confidentiality: only divulging information that has been given by a patient to the people that the patient has agreed that the information may be shared with, and not sharing the information beyond this group. It is a cornerstone of nursing practice.

confirmability: the degree to which the results of a qualitative enquiry can be confirmed by others.

consent: the process of allowing people to make choices about what they do and what is done to them when they have a full understanding of the facts and are free from external pressures.

convenience sample: a sample taken from a set of individuals who are easily accessed.

credible/credibility: believable; a term used in qualitative research to suggest that the research undertaken actually answers what it set out to answer because of the quality of the way in which the research has been done.

cross-sectional studies: studies that take place within a defined period of time and are used to determine the prevalence of disease or an exposure to a disease.

data saturation: the point during the qualitative research process at which no more new data (ideas, concepts or themes) are emerging. It is at this point that the researcher is most confident that they have collected all the data they can within their sample.

deductive: refers to research that sets out to prove an existing idea or hypothesis, to explore the truthfulness of the original idea.

dependability: consistency in the data collection if more than one researcher – or data-collection method – is used.

descriptive statistics: the use of statistics to describe the frequencies and pattern of numbers within a data set.

embedded knowledge: practice knowledge that is rooted in clinical contexts as they continually adjust to new challenges in addressing healthcare needs.

embodied knowledge: personal knowledge that is rooted in a person's individual identity as they continually interact with others in performing healthcare roles.

emotional intelligence: awareness, control and communication of feelings, plus empathising with, responding to, and enabling others to express or manage their emotions appropriately.

empirical: the notion of discovering new things using the senses or, in the case of research, different methods.

essence: the nature of something.

ethnography: a qualitative research methodology concerned with how people interact in groups.

exploratory qualitative study: a study that uses qualitative methods, but does not identify a specific qualitative methodology – often called a generic qualitative study.

generalise/generalisability/generalisable/generalised: refers to the ability of the findings of a study to be extrapolated to the wider population.

generic qualitative study: a study that uses qualitative methods, but does not identify a specific qualitative methodology – often called an exploratory study.

gold standard: the best known treatment available for a condition, usually based on good research evidence.

grounded theory: a qualitative, inductive research approach used to generate theories in the area of human interactions.

homogeneous/homogeneity: the same – as in homogenised milk, which is the same consistency throughout: there is no cream at the top.

hypothesis: an idea that quantitative research sets out to prove.

inductive: refers to the process of developing a theory or hypothesis by first collecting and examining the evidence and seeing where this leads.

inferential statistics: statistics that are used to draw conclusions about the level of association between two or more variables within a study.

informative interventions: communicating skills enabling others to exercise informed choice.

intersubjectivity: shared understanding at a psychological/human level.

justice: acting fairly so that people are treated generally in the same way.

kappa statistic: used to measure the level of agreement between two or more people measuring the same thing.

longitudinal: taking place over a period of time.

mean: also called the average; the sum of all the observations in a data set divided by the number of observations.

median: the middle value of an ordered set of observations.

member checking: the process of going back to an interviewee after an interview has been interpreted to check that the interpretation represents what they said.

meta-analysis: a statistical method used to combine the result from multiple studies to provide a very robust understanding of the effect of an intervention.

methodologies/methodology: the broad approaches to research that provide the general framework of the enquiry.

methods: in the sense that they are used in this book, the specific tools used to collect data during the research process – e.g., a questionnaire.

moral distress: the distress caused when the clinical actions undertaken are at odds with what the nurse feels to be right for the patient.

non-maleficence: the ethical principle of avoiding doing harm, perhaps better thought of as 'first do no harm'.

null hypothesis: the opposite of what the researcher actually expects to find. It is stated in this way in order to aid statistical analysis and to help demonstrate management of potential bias.

paradigm(s):   in the sense that the term is applied in this book, the philosophical position that is taken within the research; sometimes called the worldview.

PERSON evaluation tool: a framework to evaluate clinical decisions using six criteria: Patient-centred; Evidence-based; Risks assessed and managed; Safe and effective delivery of care; Outcomes of care benefit the patient; Nursing and midwifery strengths and weaknesses.

person-centred care: care that is built around the care needs and wants of the individual rather than being imposed by care profesionals.

phenomenological: lived experience from which phenomena may be deduced.

phenomenology: a research methodology within qualitative research concerned with understanding the 'essence' of an experience or perceived reality from the point of view of someone experiencing the phenomenon of interest.

probability sampling: the selection of people from a large potential study population that allows everyone the same chance of being included in the study.

prospective: going forward in time.

pulse oximetry: measurement of oxygen saturation of haemoglobin in red blood cells.

purposive sampling/purposively: refers to a method of sampling within qualitative research whereby people are chosen for inclusion because they meet the purpose of the study. This means they have experience of the phenomenon being studied.

qualitative paradigm: a paradigm associated with the social and psychological sciences. People using this paradigm are interested in discovering truths about how people experience the world and why.

qualitative research: research that explores attitudes, opinions, experiences or behaviours through interviews, focus groups or observation.

quantitative paradigm: a paradigm that views the world in a conventionally scientific sense. People using this paradigm are interested in proving associations, correlations and cause and effect.

quantitative research: research that seeks to discover relationships between variables in a statistical way.

randomised controlled trial (RCT): a specific form of experiment that is used in the clinical setting in order to compare the usefulness of two or more interventions.

recall bias: occurs when individuals in a study have to rely on their memory in order to answer certain questions. Such biases are created when people who are ill, or have another reason to remember an exposure, are better at recalling events than people who are not. Last (1995) gives the example of mothers of children with leukemia being better at recalling having had X-rays while pregnant than mothers of children who are not.

reflection-in-action: thinking and learning while actively engaged in an activity (thinking on your feet).

reflection-on-action: thinking through and reflecting on an activity after the event.

reflexive/reflexivity: the conscious engagement on the part of the researcher in being open to and expressing their own biases and opinions that might affect the carrying out and interpretation of the research.

reliability/reliable: refers to whether a method of data collection or measurement will repeatedly give the same results if used by the same person more than once or by two or more people when measuring the same phenomenon.

representative: in sampling, it means that the people included in the study are broadly similar to the population (or group) that the sample is taken from.

respondent validation: see member checking.

rigour/rigorous: a term used in qualitative research that suggests that the research process has been undertaken in a well thought through, explained and transparent manner.

saturation: see data saturation.

selection bias: bias can happen as a result of an action occurring on one side of a study and not the other. If researchers were allowed to decide which participants had which intervention in a study, it is possible that they might select patients they thought would do better in the study or try harder to follow a regime; this would be called selection bias.

sham intervention: an intervention used in the control arm of a study to ensure that the treatment arm and control arm are treated in a broadly similar way.

study population: all people who fit the study inclusion/exclusion criteria.

study sample: the people who are eventually chosen for the study.

subjective experience: impact of perceived thoughts, opinions, senses and feelings as we interact with others and the environment in developing our unique personal biographies.

supportive interventions: verbal and non-verbal skills enabling others to feel respected.

synthesised member checking: member checking (see above) which may occur up to months after an interview and in which the participant may record new insights or changes in thinking about the subject discussed.

systematic review: a process by which various research papers on a topic are identified and appraised for their quality in order to synthesise a solution to a clinical problem.

tacit knowledge: subconscious basis of intuitive, subjective understanding that influences behaviour, but which is very difficult to articulate or explain (see also embodied knowledge).

thematic analysis: analysis that involves looking for recurrent patterns and themes that arise from the data.

theoretical sampling: this occurs as the researcher builds new theories and ideas from the data they have collected and tests this theory by interviewing more subjects to see if the new theory still holds true – usually, only a feature of grounded theory research. Also called 'handy sampling'.

tracheal stricture: narrowing of the trachea.

tracheostomy tube: a tube inserted into the trachea to aid breathing.

transferable/transferability: refers to how well the findings of a qualitative study might transfer to other, similar cases. This is generally regarded as having less power than generalisability.

triangulation: a technique used to increase the credibility of research by using research approaches from both research paradigms or more than one data-collection method. It helps demonstrate the accuracy of what is found in much the same way that providing a longitude and latitude reading helps pinpoint a location on a map.

validity/valid: refers to the ability of a method (or data-collection technique) to measure what it is supposed to be measuring. For example, we know that a thermometer (if placed correctly for long enough) will measure temperature, but it is not easy to be certain that a questionnaire designed to measure quality of life actually does so because it is not always easy to define what quality of life actually is.

variable: literally something that varies, such as eye colour or age. In the research sense, it refers to the thing being explored within the study.

vegetative state: a persistent coma.

verbatim: word for word – literally, as something was said.

vital signs: measurement of consciousness, temperature, respiration, pulse and blood pressure.

References

Adamson, E (2018) Helping student nurses learn the craft of compassionate care: a relational model. *Journal of Perspectives in Applied Academic Practice*, 6 (3): 91–6. Available at: www.napier.ac.uk/~/media/worktribe/output-1660486/helping-student-nurses-learn-the-craft-of-compassionate-care-a-relational-model.pdfs

Afriyie, D (2020) Effective communication between nurses and patients: an evolutionary concept analysis. *British Journal of Community Nursing*, 25 (9): 438-45. https://doi.org/10.12968/bjcn.2020.25.9.438. PMID: 32881615

Ali, M (2017) Communication skills 1: benefits of effective communication for patients. *Nursing Times* (online); 113 (12): 18–19.

Anantapong, K, Barrado-Martín, Y, Nair, P, Rait, G, Smith, CH, Moore, KJ, Manthorpe, J, Sampson, EL and Davies, N (2021) How do people living with dementia perceive eating and drinking difficulties? A qualitative study. *Age and Ageing*, 50 (5): 1820–28. Available at: https://doi.org/10.1093/ageing/afab108

Barber, C, McLaughlin, N and Wood, J (2009) Self-awareness: the key to person-centred care? in Koubel, G and Bungay, H (eds) *The Challenge of Person-Centred Care: An Interprofessional Perspective*. Basingstoke: Palgrave.

Beauchamp, TL and Childress, JF (2013) *Principles of Biomedical Ethics* (7th edn). Oxford: Oxford University Press.

Benner, P (1984) *From Novice to Expert: Excellence and Power in Clinical Nursing Practice*. Menlo Park, CA: Addison-Wesley.

Birt, L, Scott, S, Cavers, D, Campbell, C and Walter, F (2016) Member checking: a tool to enhance trustworthiness or merely a nod to validation? *Qualitative Health Research*, 26 (13): 1802–11.

Bolton, G and Delderfield, R (2018) *Reflective Practice: Writing and Professional Development* (5th edn). Los Angeles, CA: Sage.

Brechin, A (2000) Introducing critical practice, in Brechin, A, Brown, H and Eby, MA (eds) *Critical Practice in Health and Social Care*. London: Sage.

Bridges, W and Bridges, S (2017) *Managing Transitions: Making the Most of Change* (4th edn). New York: Da Capo.

Buswell, C (1998) Feeling is believing. *Nursing Standard*, 12 (23): 20.

Byers, V (2017) The challenges of leading change in health-care delivery from the front-line. *Journal of Nursing Management*, 25 (6): 449–56.

Cambridge (2018) *Cambridge Dictionary*. Available at: dictionary.cambridge.org/dictionary/english/reflexivity

Care Quality Commission (2009) Review of the involvement and action taken by health bodies in relation to the case of Baby P. London: CQC.

Carel, H (2008) *Illness*. Stocksfield: Acumen.

Carlsson-Lalloo, E, Berg, M, Mellgren, A and Rusner, M (2018) Sexuality and childbearing as it is experienced by women living with HIV in Sweden: a lifeworld phenomenological study. *International Journal of Qualitative Studies on Health and Well-being*, 13 (1): 1487760. doi: 10.1080/17482631.2018.1487760

Carper, BA (1978) Fundamental patterns of knowing in nursing. *Advances in Nursing Science*, 1 (1): 13–23.

Chambers (2014) *The Chambers Dictionary* (13th edn). Cambridge: Chambers.

Colquhoun, L, Shepherd, V and Neil, M (2019) Pain management in new amputees: a nursing perspective. *British Journal of Nursing*, 28 (10): 638–46. Available at: https://doi.org/10.12968/bjon.2019.28.10.607

Connelly, N and Seden, J (2003) What service users say about services: the implications for managers, in Henderson, J and Atkinson, D (eds) *Managing Care in Context*. London: Routledge.

Coughlan, M and Cronin, P (2017) *Doing a Literature Review in Nursing, Health and Social Care* (2nd edn). London: Sage.

Coughlan, M, Cronin, P and Ryan, F (2007) Step-by-step guide to critiquing research: Part 1: quantitative research. *British Journal of Nursing*, 16 (11): 658–63.

Crabtree, E, Brennan, E, Davis, A and Coyle, A (2016) Improving patient care through nursing engagement in evidence-based practice. *Worldviews on Evidence- Based Nursing*, 13 (2): 172–5. Available at: https://doi.org/10.1111/wvn.12126

Craig, JV and Smyth, RL (eds) (2007) *The Evidence-Based Manual for Nurses* (2nd edn). Edinburgh: Churchill Livingstone.

Creswell, JW And Creswell JD (2018) *Research Design: Qualitative, Quantitative, and Mixed Methods Approaches* (5th edn). London: Sage.

Cromwell, DM and Boynton, B (2020) *Complexity Leadership: Nursing's Role in Health Care Delivery* (3rd edn). Philadelphia, PA: Davis.

DH (Department of Health) (1989) *Working for Patients*. London: HMSO.

DH (1991) *The Patient's Charter*. London: HMSO.

DH (2000) *The NHS Plan: A Plan for Investment, A Plan for Reform*. London: HMSO.

DH (2001) *The NHS Plan*. London: HMSO.

DH (2010) *Equity and Excellence: Liberating the NHS*. London: DH.

DH (2012a) *Caring for Our Future: Reforming Care and Support*. London: DH.

DH (2012b) *NHS Patient Experience Framework*. London: HMSO.

Driscoll, J (2007) *Practising Clinical Supervision: A Reflective Approach for Healthcare Professionals* (2nd edn). Edinburgh: Bailliere Tindall.

Dubler, NN (1992) Individual advocacy as a governing principle. *Journal of Case Management*, 13: 82–6.

Elliot, P and Koubel, G (2009) What is person-centred care? in Koubel, G and Bungay, H (eds) *The Challenge of Person-centre Care: An Interprofessional Perspective.* Basingstoke: Palgrave. pp. 29–50.

Ellis, P (2012) Rights and responsibilities, in Koubel, G and Bungay, H (eds) *Rights, Risks and Responsibilities: Interprofessional Perspectives.* Basingstoke: Palgrave.

Ellis, P (2019) Ethical concepts: what does best interests actually mean? *Journal of Kidney Care*, 4 (4): 211–13.

Ellis, P (2020) *Understanding Ethics for Nursing Students* (3rd edn). London: Sage.

Ellis, P (2022a) *Understanding Research for Nursing Students* (5th edn). London: Sage.

Ellis, P (2022b) *Leadership, Management and Team Working in Nursing* (4th edn). London: Sage.

Ellis, P and Abbott, J (2015) Preparing for revalidation. *Journal of Renal Nursing*, 7 (5): 254–5.

Ellis, P and Abbott, J (2018) Applying Lewin's change model in the kidney care unit: unfreezing. *Journal of Kidney Care*, 3 (4): 259–61.

Ellis, P and Koubel, G (2009) What is person-centred care? in Koubel, G and Bungay, H (eds) *The Challenge of Person-centred Care: An Interprofessional Perspective.* Basingstoke: Palgrave Macmillan. pp. 29–50.

Engle, R, Tyler, D, Gormley, KE, Afable, MK, Curyto, K, Adjognon, OL, Parker, VA and Sullivan, JL (2017) Identifying barriers to culture change: a qualitative analysis of the obstacles to delivering resident-centered care. *Psychological Services*, 14 (3): 316–26.

Esterhuizen, P (2019) *Reflective Practice in Nursing* (4th edn). London: Sage.

Falcó-Pegueroles, A, Rodríguez-Martín, D, Ramos-Pozón, S and Zuriguel-Pérez, E (2021) Critical thinking in nursing clinical practice, education and research: from attitudes to virtue. *Nursing Philosophy*, 22 (1): e12332. Available at: https://doi.org/10.1111/nup.12332.

Friedemann Smith, C, Møller Kristensen, B, Sand Andersen, R, Ziebland, S and Nicholson, BD (2022) Building the case for the use of gut feelings in cancer referrals: perspectives of patients referred to a non-specific symptoms pathway. *British Journal of General Practice*, 72 (714): e43-e50. doi: 10.3399/BJGP.2021.0275.

Galante, J, Dufour, G, Vainre, M, Wagner, AP, Stochl, J, Benton, A, Lathia, N, Howart, E and Jones, PB (2018) A mindfulness-based intervention to increase resilience to stress in university students (the Mindful Student Study): a pragmatic randomised controlled trial. *The Lancet: Public Health*, 3 (2): e72–e81.

Ganzini, L, Goy, ER and Miller, LL (2003) Nurses' experience with hospice patients who refuse food and fluids to hasten death. *New England Journal of Medicine*, 349: 359–65.

Gerrish, K and Lathlean, J (2015) *The Research Process in Nursing* (7th edn). Oxford: Wiley-Blackwell.

Glaser, BG and Strauss, AL (1967) *The Discovery of Grounded Theory: Strategies for Qualitative Research.* Chicago: Aldine.

Goleman, D (2020) *Emotional Intelligence.* London: Bloomsbury.

González, J and Wagenaar, R (2003) *Tuning Educational Structures in Europe: Final Report Pilot Project – Phase 1.* Bilbao: University of Deusto.

Gross, R (2020) *Psychology: The Science of Mind and Behaviour* (8th edn). London: Hodder Education.

Guarinoni, M, Petrucci, C, Lancia, L, and Motta, PC (2015) The concept of care complexity: a qualitative study. *Journal of Public Health Research,* 4 (3): 588. Available at: https://doi.org/10.4081/jphr.2015.588

Hayward, J (1979) *Information: A Prescription Against Pain.* London: Royal College of Nursing.

Hennink, M and Kaiser, B (2019) Saturation in qualitative research, in Atkinson, P, Delamont, S, Cernat, A, Sakshaug, JW and Williams RA (eds) SAGE Research Methods Foundations. Available at: https://dx.doi.org/10.4135/9781526421036822322

Her Majesty's Government (2005) Mental Capacity Act 2005. Available at: www.legislation.gov.uk/ukpga/2005/9/contents

Heron, J (2001) *Helping the Client: A Creative, Practical Guide* (5th edn). London: Sage.

Holland, K and, Jenkins, J, (2019) *Applying the Roper, Logan and Tierney Model in Practice* (3rd edn). Edinburgh: Churchill Livingstone/Elsevier.

Holmes, TH and Rahe, RH (1967) The social readjustments rating scales. *Journal of Psychosomatic Research,* 11: 213–18.

Hopson, B and Adams, J (1976) *Transition: Understanding and Managing Personal Change.* London: Martin Robertson.

Humphreys, H, Kilby, L, Kudiersky, N and Copeland, R (2021) Long COVID and the role of physical activity: a qualitative study. *BMJ Open,* 11: e047632. Available at: https://doi.org/10.1136/bmjopen-2020-047632

Hussein, ME, Jakubec, SL and Osiji, J (2015) Assessing the FACTS. *The Qualitative Report,* 20 (8): 1182–4: 110. Available at: https://doi.org/10.1186/s13075-018-1608-x

Jackson, C and Ellis, P (2010) Creative thinking for whole systems working, in Standing, M (ed.) *Clinical Judgement and Decision Making in Nursing and Interprofessional Practice.* Milton Keynes: McGraw Hill.

Jasper, M (2013) *Beginning Reflective Practice* (2nd edn). Andover: Cengage.

Jolley, J (2020) *Introducing Research and Evidence-Based Practice for Nursing and Healthcare Professionals* (3rd edn). Oxford; Routledge.

Kamel, FF and Aref, MAE (2017) Staff nurses' perception toward organizational culture and its relation to innovative work behavior at critical care units. *American Journal of Nursing Science,* 6 (3): 251–60.

King's Fund (2021) The road to renewal: five priorities for health and care. London: The King's Fund. Available at: www.kingsfund.org.uk/publications/covid-19-road-renewal-health-and-care.

King's Fund (2022) The Health and Social Care Act 2022. London: The King's Fund. Available at: www.kingsfund.org.uk/projects/health-and-care-act-2022-make-sense-legislation

Kitson, A, Ahmed, LB, Harvey, G, Seers, K and Thompson, DR (1996) From research to practice: one organisational model for promoting research-based practice. *Journal of Advanced Nursing*, 23: 430–40.

Kitson, A, Harvey, G and McCormack, B (1998) Enabling the implementation of evidence-based practice: a conceptual framework. *Quality in Health Care*, 7: 149–58.

Lamiani, G, Dordoni, P and Argentero, P (2018) Value congruence and depressive symptoms among critical care clinicians: the mediating role of moral distress. *Stress and Health*, 34 (1): 135–42.

Laming, Lord (2003) The Victoria Climbié Inquiry. Available at: https://assets.publishing.service.gov.uk/government/uploads/system/uploads/attachment_data/file/273183/5730.pdf

Last, JM (1995) *A Dictionary of Epidemiology* (3rd edn). Oxford: Oxford University Press.

Leonardsen, AC, Brynhildsen, S, Hansen, MT and Grøndahl, VA (2021) Supervising students in a complex nursing practice – a focus group study in Norway. *BMC Nursing*, 20 (1): 168. doi: 10.1186/s12912-021-00693-1

Lewin, K (1947) Frontiers in group dynamics: concept, method, and reality in social science. *Human Relations*, 1: 5–42.

Lobiondo-Wood, G and Haber, J (2013) *Nursing Research: Methods, and Critical Appraisal for Evidence Based Practice* (8th edn). St Louis, MO: Mosby.

Lopez Sanguero, SJ and Andrés Collado, M (2018) Gout characteristics and its association with the presence of cardiovascular disease: a case-control study. *Annals of the Rheumatic Diseases*, 77 (664): s2.

McArthur, C, Bai, Y, Hewston, P, Giangregorio, L, Straus, S and Papaioannou, A (2021) Barriers and facilitators to implementing evidence-based guidelines in long-term care: a qualitative evidence synthesis. *Implementation Science*, 16 (1): 70. Available at: https://doi.org/10.1186/s13012-021-01140-0

McHugh SK, Lawton R, O'Hara, JK et al. (2020) Does team reflexivity impact teamwork and communication in interprofessional hospital-based healthcare teams? A systematic review and narrative synthesis. *BMJ Quality & Safety*, 29: 672–83. Available at: https://qualitysafety.bmj.com/content/29/8/672

McKibbon, KA (1998) Evidence-based practice. *Bulletin of the Medical Library Association*, 86 (3): 396–401.

Meads, G, Barr, H, Scott, R, Ashcroft, J and Wild, A (2005) *The Case for Inter-Professional Collaboration*. Oxford: Blackwell.

Medicines and Healthcare Products Regulatory Agency (2021) Patient involvement strategy 2021–5. Available at: https://assets.publishing.service.gov.uk/government/uploads/system/uploads/attachment_data/file/1022370/Patient_involvement_strategy.pdf

Merritt, RK, Hotham, S, Hotham, GL and Schrag, A (2018) The subjective experience of Parkinson's disease: a qualitative study in 60 people with mild to moderate Parkinson's in 11 European countries. *European Journal of Person Centered Healthcare*, 6 (3). Available at: https://kar.kent.ac.uk/id/eprint/67120

Moule, P (2021) *Making Sense of Research in Nursing, Health and Social Care* (7th edn). London: Sage.

Neil, MJE, (2016) Pain after amputation. *British Journal of Anaesthesia Education*, 16 (3): 107–12. Available at: https://doi.org/10.1093/bjaed/mkv028

NHS (2019) The long term NHS plan: a summary. Available at: www.longtermplan.nhs.uk/wp-content/uploads/2019/01/the-nhs-long-term-plan-summary.pdf

Natuhwera, G, Ellis, P and Acuda, SW (2021) Women's lived experiences of advanced cervical cancer: a descriptive qualitative study. *International Journal of Palliative Nursing*, 27 (9): 334–47.

NICE (2011) 2010/2011 review. London: NICE. Available at: http://review2010-2011.nice.org.uk/patients_public/index.html

NICE (2013) Patient and public involvement policy. London: NICE. Available at: www.nice.org.uk/media/default/About/NICE-Communities/Public-involvement/Patient-and-public-involvement-policy/Patient-and-public-involvement-policy-November-2013.pdf

NICE (2018) Principles for putting evidence-based guidance into practice. London: NICE. Available at: www.nice.org.uk/Media/Default/About/what-we-do/Into-practice/Principles-for-putting-evidence-based-guidance-into-practice.pdf

NICE (2020) Decision making and mental capacity: Quality standard (QS194). Available at: www.nice.org.uk/guidance/qs194/chapter/Quality-statement-4-Best-interests-decision-making

NICE (2021) COVID-19 rapid guideline: managing COVID-19 (NG191). London: NICE.

NICE (2022) Epilepsies in children, young people and adults. NICE guideline [NG217]. London: NICE. Available at: www.nice.org/uk/guidance/ng217

NMC (2018a) *Future Nurse: Standards of Proficiency for Registered Nurses*. London: NMC.

NMC (2018b) *The Code: Professional Standards of Practice and Behaviour for Nurses, Midwives and Nursing Associates*. London: NMC.

NMC (2019) *Guidance on Health and Character*. London: NMC.

Olsson, A, Thunborg, C, Björkman, A, Blom, A, Sjöberg, F, Salzmann-Erikson, M (2020) A scoping review of complexity science in nursing. *Journal of Advanced Nursing*, 76: 1961–76. doi: 10.1111/jan.14382

OPSI (Office of Public Sector Information) (1989) The Children Act 1989. London: OPSI. Available at: www.opsi.gov.uk/acts/acts1989/ukpga_19890041_en_1

OPSI (Office of Public Sector Information) (2018) The Data Protection Act 2018. London: OPSI. Available at: www.legislation.gov.uk/ukpga/2018/12/contents/enacted

Otham, SY and El-hady, MM (2015) Effect of implementing structured communication messages on the clinical outcomes of unconscious patients. *Journal of Nursing Education and Practice*, 3 (9): 117–31.

Parahoo, K (2014) *Nursing Research: Principles, Process and Issues* (3rd edn). London: Palgrave Macmillan.

Patients Association (2020) Being a patient: first report of the Patients Association's patient experience programme – executive summary. Harrow: The Patients Association. Available at www.patients-association.org.uk/Handlers/Download.ashx?IDMF=2898fa05-69fa-4e66-b856-c150080d432c.

Pearson, B (2017) The clinical governance of multidisciplinary care. *International Journal of Health Governance*, 22 (4): 246–50. Available at: https://doi.org/10.1108/IJHG-03-2017-0007.

Petticrew, M and Roberts, H (2003) Evidence, hierarchies and typologies: horses for courses. *Journal of Epidemiology and Community Health*, 57 (7): 527–9.

Pijl-Zieber, EM, Barton, S, Konkin, J and Awosoga, O (2015) Disconnects in pedagogy and practice in community health nursing clinical experiences: qualitative findings of a mixed method study. *Nurse Education Today*, 35 (10): e43–8.

Polit, DF and Tatano Beck, C (2020) *Essentials of Nursing Research: Appraising Evidence for Nursing Practice* (10th edn). London: Lippincott, Williams & Wilkins.

Pope, C and Mays, N (2020) *Qualitative Research in Health Care* (4th edn). London: Wiley Blackwell.

Price, B (2021) *Critical Thinking & Writing in Nursing* (5th edn). London: Learning Matters/Sage.

Reeves, S, Pelone, F, Harrison, R, Goldman, J and Zwarenstein, M (2017) Interprofessional collaboration to improve professional practice and healthcare outcomes. *Cochrane Database of Systematic Reviews*. 6: CD000072. Available at: https://doi.org/10.1002/14651858.CD000072.pub3.

Reinharz, S (1997) Who am I? The need for a variety of selves in the field, in Hertz, R (ed.) *Reflexivity and Voice*. Thousand Oaks, CA: Sage.

Rodgers, S (1994) An exploratory study of research utilization by nurses in general medical and surgical wards. *Journal of Advanced Nursing*, 20: 904–11.

Roets-Merken, LM, Zuidema, SU, Vernooij-Dassen, MJFJ, Teerenstra, S, Hermsen, PGJM, Kempen, GIJM and Graff, MJL (2018) Effectiveness of a nurse-supported self-management programme for dual sensory impaired older adults in long-term care: a cluster randomised controlled trial. *BMJ Open*, 8 (1): e016674. doi: 10.1136/bmjopen-2017-016674

Rogers, EM (1962) *Diffusion of Innovations.* Glencoe: Free Press.

Rogers, M (2013) *Daniel Pelka Serious Case Review, Coventry LSCB.* Available at: www.lgiu. org.uk/wp-content/uploads/2013/10/Daniel-Pelka-Serious-Case-Review-Coventry-LSCB.pdf

Roper, N, Logan, WW and Tierney, AJ (2000) *The Roper–Logan–Tierney Model of Nursing: Based on Activities of Living.* Edinburgh: Churchill Livingstone.

Sackett, DL, Rosenberg, WM, Gray, JA, Haynes, RB and Richardson, WS (1996) Evidence-based medicine: what it is and what it isn't. *British Medical Journal,* 312 (7023): 71–2.

Schmidt, FL and Hunter, JE (2015) *Methods of Meta-Analysis: Correcting Error and Bias in Research Findings* (3rd edn). New York: Sage.

Scholtes, P (1998) *The Leader's Handbook: Making Things Happen, Getting Things Done.* New York: McGraw Hill.

Schön, DA (1983) *The Reflective Practitioner.* New York: Basic Books.

Sennett, R (2008) *The Craftsman.* London: Allen Lane/Penguin Books.

Sitzia, J, Cotterell, P and Richardson, A (2004) *Formative Evaluation of the Cancer Partnership Project.* London: Macmillan Cancer Relief.

Skilton, AM, Low, LG and Dimaras, H (2020) Patients, public and service users are experts by experience: an overview from ophthalmology research in Canada, UK and Beyond. *Ophthalmology and Therapy,* 9: 207–13. Available at: https://doi.org/10.1007/s40123-020-00237-x

Smith, S, Gentleman, M, Loads, D and Pullin, S (2014) An exploration of a restorative space: a creative approach to reflection for nurse lecturers focused on experiences of compassion in the workplace. *Nurse Education Today,* 34 (9): 1225–31.

Sousa, H, Frontini, R, Ribeiro, O, Paúl, C, Costa, E, Amado, L, Miranda, V, Ribeiro, F and Figueiredo, D (2022) Caring for patients with end-stage renal disease during COVID-19 lockdown: What (additional) challenges to family caregivers? *Scandinavian Journal of Caring Sciences,* 36 (1): 215–24. Available at: https://doi.org/10.1111/scs.12980

Standing, M (2007) Clinical decision-making skills on the developmental journey from student to registered nurse: a longitudinal inquiry. *Journal of Advanced Nursing,* 60 (3): 257–69.

Standing, M (2010) Perceptions of clinical decision-making: a matrix model, in Standing, M (ed.) *Clinical Judgement and Decision-Making: Nursing and Interprofessional Healthcare.* Maidenhead: Open University Press.

Standing, M (2020) *Clinical Judgement and Decision-Making for Nursing Students* (4th edn). London: Sage.

Stängle, S, Schnepp, W and Fringer, A (2019) The need to distinguish between different forms of oral nutrition refusal and different forms of voluntary stopping of eating and drinking. *Palliative Care and Social Practice,* 13. Available at: https://journals.sagepub.com/doi/full/10.1177/1178224219875738

Steglitz, J, Warnick, J, Hoffman, SA, Johnston, WD and Spring, B (2015) Evidence-based practice. *International Encyclopedia of the Social and Behavioral Sciences.* doi: 10.1016/B978-0-08-097086-8.10540-9

Straus, SE, Galziou, P, Richardson, W and Haynes, RB (2010) *Evidence-based Medicine: How to Practise and Teach EBM* (4th edn). New York: Churchill Livingstone.

Sundberg, LR, Garvare, R and Nyström, ME (2017) Reaching beyond the review of research evidence: a qualitative study of decision making during the development of clinical practice guidelines for disease prevention in healthcare. *BMC Health Service Research*, 17 (344). Available at: https://doi.org/10.1186/s12913-017-2277-1

Tamunomiebi, M and Uhuru, G (2018) Group, teams and tasks in the organization: a historical escortion. *European Journal of Business and Management Research*, 3 (4). Available at: https://doi.org/doi: 10.24018/ejbmr.2018.3.4.15

Thorne, S (2020) Rethinking Carper's personal knowing for 21st century nursing. *Nursing Philosophy*, 21: e12307. Available at: https://doi.org/10.1111/nup.12307.

van Draanen, J (2017) Introducing reflexivity to evaluation practice. *American Journal of Evaluation*, 38 (3): 360–75. doi: 10.1177/1098214016668401

Warren, CE, Njue, R, Ndwiga, C and Abuya, T (2017) Manifestations and drivers of mistreatment of women during childbirth in Kenya: implications for measurement and developing interventions. *Pregnancy and Childbirth*, 17: 102. Available at: https://doi.org/10.1186/s12884-017-1288-6

Weisbeck, S, Lind, C and Ginn, C (2019) Patient empowerment: an evolutionary concept analysis. *International Journal of Caring Sciences*, 12 (2): 1148–55.

West Sussex Adults Safeguarding Board (2014) Orchid View: serious case review. Available at: www.hampshiresab.org.uk/wp-content/uploads/June-2014-Orchid-View-Serious-Case-Review-Report.pdf

Wilson, B, Woodlands, A and Barrettt, D (2018) *Care Planning: A Guide for Nurses* (3rd edn). Abingdon: Routledge.

Yoder, LH, Cengiz, A, Hinkley, T, Hertel, RA, Gallagher-Ford, L and Koshy Thomas, B (2022) Medical-surgical nurses' EBP beliefs and competencies. *Worldviews on Evidence-Based Nursing*, 19 (2): 149–59. Available at: https://doi.org/10.1111/wvn.12567

Yoost, BL and Crawford, LR (2022) *Fundamentals of Nursing: Active Learning for Collaborative Practice* (3rd edn). St Louis: Elsevier.

Index